Stress

Marietta Whittlesey

American Family Health Institute™

Medical Board

Stanley J. Dudrick, MD
Clinical Professor of Surgery
University of Texas Medical School, Houston, Texas

Jo Eland, RN, PhD
Assistant Professor, University of Iowa
Iowa City, Iowa

Dennis E. Leavelle, MD
Consulting Pathologist, Department of Laboratory Medicine
Mayo Clinic, Rochester, Minnesota

Julena Lind, MN, RN
Director of Education, Center for Health Information, Education and Research
at California Medical Center, Los Angeles, California

Ara G. Paul, PhD
Dean, College of Pharmacy, University of Michigan
Ann Arbor, Michigan

Richard Payne, MD
Clinical Assistant Neurologist, Memorial Sloan-Kettering Cancer Center
New York, New York

William R. Truscott, MD
Diplomate, American Academy of Family Practice, Lansdale Medical Group
Lansdale, Pennsylvania

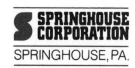

SPRINGHOUSE CORPORATION
SPRINGHOUSE, PA.

The charter of the American Family Health Institute is to research and produce high-quality publications that enhance the health of individuals and their families. Essential to health are physical, emotional, and social well-being, not just the absence of illness or infirmity. The Institute's Medical Board has produced the *Health and Fitness* books to share up-to-date and authoritative information that can give readers greater personal control over their health maintenance.

Library of Congress Cataloging-in-
Publication Data
Whittlesey, Marietta
   Stress.

   (Health and fitness series)
   Includes index.
   1. Stress (Psychology).   2. Stress
(Physiology). I. Brunner, Lillian Sholtis.
II. American Family Health Institute. Medical
Board. III. Title. IV. Series.   [DNLM:
1. Stress—popular works.   2. Stress,
Psychological—popular works.   QZ 160
W627s]
BF575.S75W48   1986   158'.1   85-30264
ISBN 0-87434-023-3

The procedures and explanations given in this publication are based on research and consultation with medical and nursing authorities. To the best of our knowledge, these procedures and explanations reflect currently accepted medical practice; nevertheless, they can't be considered absolute and universal recommendations. For individual application, treatment suggestions must be considered in light of the individual's health, subject to a doctor's specific recommendations. The authors and the publisher disclaim responsibility for any adverse effects resulting directly or indirectly from the suggested procedures, from any undetected errors, or from the reader's misunderstanding of the text.

Contents

Stress

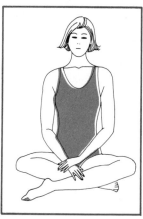

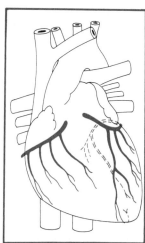

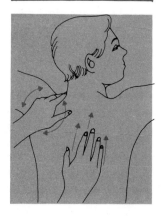

1

What stress is

Adrenal glands

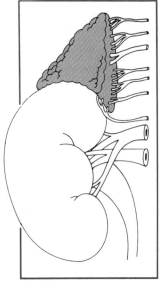

This drawing shows the adrenal gland's position on top of the kidney. (You have two kidneys and two adrenals.) Each adrenal's upper section is called the cortex; the lower section, the medulla. The cortex produces hormones called corticoids. One type of corticoid regulates mineral and water balance, blood pressure, and protein and carbohydrate metabolism. Another corticoid regulates your immune system's response to illness or injury.

The medulla secretes the hormone adrenaline, which helps you mobilize for fight or flight.

- "Sometimes I feel like I can't go on. I can't cope with my life any longer."
- "I feel tired all the time, even after I've had a good night's sleep."
- "I've been getting a headache that comes on in the middle of the day, and nothing seems to make it go away."
- "I feel depressed and drained, and I don't know why."
- "I've been fighting a lot with my spouse over unimportant things."
- "I never seem to have enough time to do all the things people expect me to do."
- "I can't concentrate."
- "I don't feel like I'm in control of my life, and I don't like it."
- "I can't stop eating."
- "I fly off the handle very easily."
- "I've been grinding my teeth at night."
- "I seem to have a lot of colds."
- "I'm bothered by back pain that just won't go away, but my doctor can't find any reason for it."
- "I smoke cigarettes, and I know it's unhealthy, but I can't quit."

Sound familiar? Feelings and symptoms like these are common occurrences for many of us. If they're part of your life, chances are you're suffering from the effects of stress.

We live in a stressful world, and although a certain amount of stress keeps us on our toes, more stress than we can handle has the opposite effect. Too much stress can make us feel our worst and, if continued too long, can even cause us to become ill—unless we learn some simple facts about identifying and coping with events, people, or things that cause stress in our lives. This book will help you understand what stress is, how it can make you sick, and what you can do about stress before it hurts you.

An overview

Stress is your body's response to any demand made upon it. That means pleasant and unpleasant events can stress you. Think about taking a vacation trip, for example. Wonderful as getting away may be, all the last-minute preparations will probably make you rush, building up stress. This response is normal until it gets out of hand. Controlling stress, then, means adapting and changing as circumstances demand.

Just being sick

We hear the word *stress* so often that most of us think we know what stress is. The concept of stress was introduced to medicine by Dr. Hans Selye, an Austrian-born doctor working in Canada. In the mid-1920s, Selye became interested in the similarities among various very different diseases and conditions. He noted that whether a patient was suffering from an injury, cancer, or an infectious disease such as hepatitis, he or she shared certain underlying characteristics in common with all other patients. These common signs included weight loss, apathy, lack of appetite, and a general lack of strength. Dr. Selye called these symptoms the syndrome of "just being sick."

When Dr. Selye explored this syndrome of "just being sick" in greater detail, he found that other things as well as illness can cause this syndrome. Many different types of good and bad life events and even thoughts and emotions can cause this feeling of "just being sick." When we're undergoing changes—whether they're physical or emotional, good or bad—our bodies go through certain predictable changes. Sometimes we're not even aware of these changes. If these internal changes continue, some weak link in our bodies will break down eventually, and we'll become sick. This is why getting married or buying a new home can be as stressful as getting divorced or staying in a bad job. "Stress," explains Dr. Selye, "is the nonspecific response of the body to any demand made upon it." All the different good and bad events and feelings that we have mentioned have one thing in common: they force you to get used to something new, to adapt. We're all constantly adapting to new things, things we like and things we don't like. This adaptation isn't harmful; it's part of being alive.

Fight or flight

"After our two cars collided, I'll never forget the feeling I had as I realized that my two children were still in the back seat of that crumpled wreckage. Broken glass was everywhere. The other car involved had already burst into flames, and I was terrified that mine was about to also. I could hear little Brian whimpering as though he were badly injured, but from the baby came an ominous silence. To this day I have no idea how I did it (I'm only five feet tall and weigh under a hundred pounds), but I got that crumpled door open, and I man-

Stressors
The events and circum-
stances that create stress
are called stressors.

aged to get them out of the car. The whole thing took less than a minute. I was just flooded with this super-human strength as though I could pick up that whole car, if I needed to, to get my babies out safely."

How can this feat of strength be explained? It's a survival response we all have within us that dates back to our earliest ancestors. In fact, we share it with animals.

The physiology of stress

As his work proceeded, Dr. Selye noted that whatever caused the stress—infection, excessive heat, extreme fatigue—the body produced the same cluster of internal changes. The adrenals enlarged, the thymus gland and various lymph nodes shrank, and eventually ulcers appeared in the stomach and small intestine.

Your lymph nodes function as part of the immune system. Their job is to strain invading particles out of your blood. Major lymph nodes are in your armpits and groin and along the sides of your neck. When you have a cold and have "swollen glands," you're feeling the lymph nodes under your jaw.

The pituitary's link to the adrenals

Brain

Pituitary gland

Nerve impulses

Adrenal glands

Kidneys

Major clusters of lymph nodes

Your body's response to stress

When you're threatened, your hypothalamus, a part of your brain that controls emotions and basic drives such as hunger and thirst, sends signals to your adrenal gland and to the pituitary. These signals say: "Mobilize! Get ready to fight or run for it!".The adrenals secrete adrenalin and other substances that prepare you to fight or flee or to repair damages to your body that may occur as you defend yourself. You've probably felt your adrenal response: your heart beats faster, you feel a rush of energy, your blood flow increases. At the same time, blood is redirected from your skin and stomach to your muscles, where it may be needed for fight or flight. Fats and sugars are released into your bloodstream for quick energy, and other released substances help your blood clot more quickly in case you're injured.

It's called the "fight or flight" response. A cat arching its back and hissing at a dog also illustrates a fight or flight response. The cat's body goes through the same internal reactions yours does when something threatens you. The reactions in the cat's body ready it to fight the dog or to flee. The fight or flight response prepared our earliest ancestors to fight or escape from life-threatening situations. This response is involuntary—we can't ordinarily control it.

This strong fight or flight response was very useful millions of years ago. Our prehistoric ancestors faced life-threatening situations just about every day. Finding food was a source of stress, as was contending with the animals that considered human beings food. Sometimes people fought such animals, and sometimes they decided to flee. The ability quickly to decide what to do was essential to survival.

Nowadays, life isn't that dangerous for most of us. Even so, we still make use of the prehistoric fight or flight response. And that's not usually a good thing. A full-blown fight or flight response to the minor annoyances of daily life harms more than it helps. Certainly, if you're attacked by a mugger or if you're engaged in an athletic competition, your body's ability to mobilize itself on the spot can be important. But for most of us, most of the time, such a response is too much. We're no longer fighting for our lives, but our bodies act as though we were. Society has changed and is still changing, but our bodies haven't had a chance to keep pace. We're living inside bodies designed to hunt mastodons for food and to battle enemy tribes, though most of us have little call for such abilities. The result is that we overreact to the frequent but hardly life-threatening stressors of daily life with a massive mobilization. Noise, arguments, missed deadlines, a new baby—any situation that requires us to adapt—all provoke some degree of fight or flight response and end up causing our bodies to pump up a lot of stress hormones designed to get us out of a real emergency. The driver behind you honks his horn, the baby throws her cereal on the floor, you accept a marriage proposal; and your body may act as though you had been jumped by a mountain lion. Some of us compound the problem by being especially sensitive: we're more likely to respond to everyday annoyances with a full-

What your body does during vigilance

The chronic "on guard" response is somewhat different from the short-term fight or flight response. The hypothalamus stimulates the pituitary to put out adrenocorticotropic hormone, or ACTH. This medical mouthful is a hormone that signals the adrenal cortex to release cortisol. Cortisol causes you to retain more salt, thereby increasing your blood pressure. It also enhances the clotting ability of your blood so that you won't lose as much blood if you're injured. Interestingly, the vigilance response causes a drop in the production of sex hormones so you'll retain more energy to survive the stress. Cortisol and the other anti-inflammatory corticoids lower the activity of the immune system and decrease disease resistance. Just as the fight or flight response developed for coping with emergencies, the vigilance response developed for coping with long-term survival threats like food deprivation or survival in intense cold. But the chronic elevation of cortisol can give way to high blood pressure as well as to the depression and apathy often associated with prolonged stress.

blown fight or flight response than to shrug them off in some way.

If the fight or flight response is evoked scores of times each day, your body is doing repeatedly what it was designed to do only in emergencies. As we'll see, chronic stress with no way of releasing it plays an important part in some, if not most, of the diseases that plague us. This overzealous alarm reaction can be far worse than the minor annoyance that evoked it, and we must learn to tone down our responses in these situations. On the other hand, when the stressor is real—invading viruses or danger in our path—we want the response to be as strong and swift as possible.

The vigilance response

The medical intern working 36-hour shifts, the fire warden in his tower, the air traffic controller guiding in passenger jets...What do all these people have in common? They're relying on another type of stress response that their bodies have in order to pull through the almost continuous stresses that they're enduring. Whereas the fight or flight response is a short-term response to on-the-spot stress, our bodies are also capable of responding to a long-term threat, digging in for prolonged survival under negative conditions. According to Dr. Robert Eliot, director of the National Center of Preventive and Stress Medicine in Phoenix and author of *Is It Worth Dying For?*, this vigilance response, as he calls it, is "the chronic response to loss of control." The person fighting an illness, the student studying for an important exam, the soldier guarding a camp are all using their vigilance responses.

In ancient times, people usually did end up fighting or fleeing and so worked off the adrenalin and other hormones that they produced. Today, we usually don't have the opportunity to fight or flee, but instead have to swallow our emotions in the name of good manners and acting civilized. Furthermore, many of us now lead mostly sedentary lives. We no longer work on the farm or engage in heavy labor, the sort of hard physical activity that provides an excellent outlet for all the fight or flight hormones that get pumped up. Many of us wisely use exercise as a release of our stress, thus avoiding undue strain on our hearts, our circulatory systems, our muscles, and numerous other body parts.

Stress and the physical fitness boom

Our need to work off the stress hormones that we're constantly churning up may be one of the reasons for the great popularity of exercise in America today. As we expend less physical energy on day-to-day survival, we're finding that we need to stay fit in other ways. Keeping our bodies in top shape is a very important way to keep the stesses of everyday life from harming us. Regular exercise helps strengthen the heart and lungs, making them more efficient at their jobs. Most experts advise regular exercise for at least 20 minutes, three times a week. Aerobic exercises like walking, running and biking are all excellent for releasing tension.

Aerobic exercises

Diminished stress is only one of the many benefits of regular exercise. Because they raise your heart rate, aerobic exercises are the most beneficial kind of exercises. For the best effects of aerobic exercises, you must work a little harder than what is comfortable for you but a lot less harder than all-out exertion. This level is called your aerobic training level. The easiest way to find your aerobic training level is to take your pulse during exercise. When your heart is beating at between 70 and 85 percent of its maximum rate, you'll be working at the right level.

This chart is designed to help you determine your aerobic training level. To use this chart, find your age in the left column and read across to find your 70 and 85 percent maximum pulse rates during a 10-second reading.

For the most beneficial results, maintain your pulse during exercise between the 70 and 85 percent figures.

If you want to know what your 1-minute pulse rate should be, multiply your 10-second count by 6.

Target 10-second pulse rates by age

Age	70 percent	85 percent
20	23	28
25	23	28
30	22	27
35	22	26
40	21	26
45	20	25
50	20	24
55	19	23
60	19	23
65	18	22
70	18	21

Questions and answers about stress

Q: What's the difference between the stress syndrome and the fight or flight response?
A: The fight or flight response is the first stage of the stress syndrome. Dr. Selye said that the stress syndrome (or the "general adaptation syndrome" as he first called it) occurs in three phases:

• The stage of alarm, in which your body mobilizes itself to cope with the stressor.
• The stage of resistance, in which your body actively resists the stressor—for instance, by sending immune system soldiers to fight an infection.
• The stage of exhaustion, in which your body, or whatever part of it is under stress, can no longer resist the stressor and gives out.

The stage of alarm and the fight or flight response are basically the same, and the vigilance response and the stage of resistance also basically correspond to each other.

Q: When do we reach the stage of exhaustion?
A: We don't always or even usually reach this final stage of the stress response. If our bodies are successful in resisting the stress, exhaustion doesn't come. We adapt to the stressor instead and make whatever adjustments are needed for this adaptation. This is true both for physical stress and for psychological stress. For instance, using your muscles unusually hard for a prolonged period of running is stressful to your body and may bring you close to a state of physical exhaustion. As you train, your body adapts to the increased demands of running, and you'll take longer and longer to reach the exhaustion point.

When we're talking about psychological stress, the stage of exhaustion corresponds to that stage of final burnout where we feel we can no longer cope. Then we tend to fall prey to various illnesses. Most of us will withstand prolonged stress before we reach this point, and we'll receive numerous warnings along the way that the body is having problems coping with the stress that we're under. These warning symptoms might include chronic headaches, sleep problems, or irritability. They mean that we should slow down before we reach the state of psychological exhaustion that can cause both physical and emotional illness.

2

Are you under stress?

Which of these people is suffering from the effects of stress?

• Alice, age 15, is studying for a math exam that's very important for her to pass. She knows that if she doesn't, she'll have to go to summer school and miss a visit to the Grand Canyon with her parents.

• Juan Correa can't remember feeling happier. In two hours he'll be married to the most beautiful girl in the world.

• Betty and Jack Braverman are sharing a last cup of coffee on the porch of their old house. In a few minutes, the movers will take their furniture to their beautiful and much larger new home.

• As she tries to keep a stiff upper lip throughout the funeral service, Mrs. O'Keefe can't help wondering how she and the children will manage without Mr. O'Keefe.

If you said that Alice and Mrs. O'Keefe are stressed, you're correct, but Juan Correa and the Bravermans are also experiencing stress. To understand why, consider Dr. Selye's original definition of stress as "the rate of wear and tear in the body." Stress is really the body's response to changes. New situations that require adaptation initially trigger the output of the adrenal stress hormones.

Your first day on a new job is stressful, and your body responds with some degree of stress response. Your mouth may be dry, you may be fidgety, and you may perspire more than normal. If you're able to adapt to the new job successfully, the stress you experience continually decreases until just going to work doesn't require adaptation energy. Of course, if you're expecting a hard day, if you've begun to hate the job, or if you have a new boss, you'll again experience some degree of physiological response.

A wedding or the birth of a child is a joyous event, but you respond to both with a fight or flight response.

Stress, then, may occur with both good and bad life events. Change and the stress it brings are necessary for growth and even for the continuance of life. Con-

The happiest day of your life

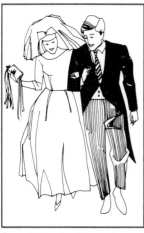

A wedding day is one for happiness, but don't be surprised if that happiness causes stress. Stress can occur with both good and bad life events, so the happiest day of your life may well be one of the most stressful.

Hardiness

In a study of heavy smokers, those who developed lung cancer over the course of the five-year study had about the same number of major life changes as those who stayed healthy. The difference between the smokers who got cancer and those who didn't? The cancer patients perceived these life changes as more stressful, and they blamed themselves more for the changes. (This study doesn't suggest that smoking, even with the right attitude, is safe. Smoking is dangerous to everyone.)

stantly thinking of how much stress you're under is stressful in itself. Stress couldn't be avoided even if that were possible or desirable. As Dr. Selye points out, "Complete freedom from stress is death."

Our stress response enables us to try new things and to face the stages and experiences of life, both the good and the bad, that we all must live through. We can react to these stressors with the development of new strengths and potentials as well as with the development of diseases. So instead of avoiding stress, we must aim to reduce unnecessary stressors in our lives and to reduce our physiological response to them.

The Holmes and Rahe life events scale

Have you ever noticed how you or others tend to get sick around the time of major life events? The bride develops fever blisters the morning of her wedding, the widower suffers a heart attack two months after his wife's death, the new parents get the flu. Several psychiatrists also noted these "coincidences" and began to keep detailed biographical and medical histories of thousands of patients. They found that major illnesses such as heart disease, ulcers, and psychiatric problems often occurred after major life changes. (This may happen because stress seems generally to weaken the immune system and decrease resistance to illness. Certain stressors or our responses to them may cause such specific changes as an increase in cholesterol in the blood or an increase in stomach acid secretion.)

Out of these observations about the timing of life events and major illness came the Holmes and Rahe Social Readjustment Scale, devised in 1967 by Thomas H. Holmes, MD, and Richard H. Rahe, MD, at the University of Washington School of Medicine. This scale lists important life changes ranging in severity from death of a spouse to minor violations of the law. Each life change is assigned a value according to the magnitude of the adaptation response it evokes. Thus, the death of a spouse is four times harder to adjust to than beginning or ending school.

The social readjustment rating scale

The Holmes and Rahe Social Readjustment Scale has been reprinted here to help you assess how much life change you're asking yourself to adapt to and how it may affect your health over the next couple of years.

The social readjustment rating scale

Event	Rating	Your Score
Death of spouse	100	____
Divorce	73	____
Marital separation	65	____
Jail term	63	____
Death of close family member	63	____
Personal injury or illness	53	____
Marriage	50	____
Fired from work	47	____
Marital reconciliation	45	____
Retirement	45	____
Change in health of family member	44	____
Pregnancy	40	____
Sex difficulties	39	____
Gain of new family member	39	____
Business readjustment	39	____
Change in financial state	38	____
Death of close friend	37	____
Change to different line of work	36	____
Change in number of arguments with spouse	35	____
New mortgage	31	____
Foreclosure of mortgage or loan	30	____
Change in responsibilities at work	29	____
Son or daughter leaving home	29	____
Trouble with in-laws	29	____
Outstanding personal achievement	28	____
Spouse begins or stops work	26	____
Begin or end school	26	____
Change in living conditions	25	____
Revision of personal habits	24	____
Trouble with boss	23	____
Change in work hours or conditions	20	____
Change in residence	20	____
Change in school	20	____
Change in recreation	19	____
Change in religious commitment	19	____
Change in social activities	18	____
Small mortgage or loan	17	____
Change in sleeping habits	16	____
Change in number of family get-togethers	15	____
Change in eating habits	15	____
Vacation	13	____
Christmas/Hanukkah/New Year's	12	____
Minor violations of the law	11	____
	Your total	____

Go down the list of items and circle those events that have occurred over the past year. Then add up your score. While this quiz can't tell your present state of health or whether you'll react to major life events by becoming ill, it can give you a rough idea of the major stress elements in your life during the last year.

Your score	Evaluating your score
150 or below	You don't have a greatly increased risk of serious illness. Your chances of developing an illness in the next two years is about one in three.
150 to 300	Your chances of becoming seriously ill in the next two years are higher than they might be if you were under less stress. Since a lot is going on in your life, remember to take extra care of yourself so that your body doesn't become exhausted trying to adjust. Be sure to eat well, get plenty of rest and exercise, and don't neglect to take some time out for yourself.
300 +	A score of 300 or more indicates that you're living through a lot of life changes and run a higher risk of becoming ill over the next couple of years. Read on to see how you might either reduce the number of stressful changes that you're living through or how you might at least reduce your body's reaction to them. Again, don't forget the importance of proper diet, rest, and exercise in keeping your body fit and able to resist any problems brought on by stress.

Stress build-up *Stress usually accumulates, an event at a time. This chart shows the major stressful events during 6 months in Nancy Marble's life, their Holmes-Rahe values, and what the stress may mean for Nancy Marble.*	Death of a sister	Arguments with spouse	Sex difficulties
	(63)	(35)	(39)

Control and stress
Having some control over events helps you reduce stress, but recognizing what you can't control and letting it go can also reduce stress.

Coping with stress

Using the Holmes and Rahe scale, let's look at a year in the life of Nancy Marble, a 58-year-old social studies teacher. Mrs. Marble's year began with the death of her sister (a stress rating of 63). Later in the spring, her husband, George, passed his seventieth birthday and went into company-imposed retirement. His difficulties in adjusting to retirement caused the Marbles to argue bitterly and often—something new to their happy thirty-five-year marriage (a rating of 35). The increased arguments put a major damper on what had been a satisfying sexual relationship (39). In order to help George readjust, the Marbles greatly increased the number of parties they gave and attended (18). Although Nancy didn't say anything about it to her husband, this increased socializing put a strain on her. She wasn't a drinker, and somehow the cheerful revels of the other new retirees and their spouses bored and depressed her. She would have preferred more time to do what she enjoyed: reading, bird watching, and planning her class time. Things came to a head in the chaotic Christmas season (12) when Mrs. Marble was stopped for speeding through a red light to get to the supermarket before it closed for the holiday (11). As the police officer wrote out her ticket, Nancy put her head down on the steering wheel and burst into tears.

Nancy Marble's total score is 178. Thus, according to Holmes and Rahe, she has about even chances of developing an illness or staying well over the next two years. Let's see how Nancy might stack the odds more in her favor and stay well.

Timing of those life events over which we have some control is a major key to keeping life's changes from using up too much adaptation energy all at once and

Change in social activities	Holiday demands	Minor law violation	Total	
(18)	(12)	(11)	(178)	Higher than normal chance of serious sickness

Planning can reduce stress

Several studies by psychologists have shown that planning ahead may reduce any adverse effects on health brought about by predictable life changes such as retirement. Many companies have responded to this information in a very positive fashion by running helpful pre-retirement seminars and discussion groups. If your company hasn't such a plan, you may be able to make your own arrangements. For example, one thirty-year employee of a college continued his association after retirement by giving tours of the campus two days a week. Talking about this later, he said he felt this continuing sense of connection with "the old place" kept him feeling useful. For some people, this tapering-off period is the time to develop new interests or devote more time to hobbies.

On the other hand, some people think of retirement as a highly deserved rest period when they don't even want to think of doing anything more ambitious than lying in a hammock with a cool drink.

overwhelming our adaptive mechanism. Learning not to try to control things we realistically can't control is equally important as a stress management tool.

Mrs. Marble had no control over her sister's death, but she could control her response to it. Instead of keeping a stiff upper lip and throwing herself into her work, Nancy Marble might have done better to talk about her grief to her family and friends, her clergyman, or a health professional such as a doctor or a counselor. That she single-handedly put her sister's affairs in order according to her sister's wishes and got her apartment on the market helped. Doing these essential tasks gave her a sense of taking charge and coping, and this, as we'll see, is a powerful stress reducer for a take-charge person like Nancy Marble.

Some people are happy when they retire. They've been looking forward to a well-earned rest for many years, and their retirement is all that they dreamed it would be. Others, like George Marble, aren't so lucky. Although they may not have enjoyed going in to work day after day, year after year, when the time comes to leave their job, they suffer from a real sense of depression. The Marbles could have lessened George's sense of loss and depression by planning ahead for a gradual transition.

Marital quarrels

Marital quarrels that serve only to vent anger solve nothing and perpetuate stress. However, marital quarrels that solve problems are sometimes worth the stress they cause.

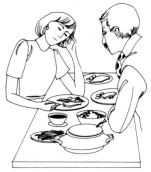

Devising strategies

Usually, you need a mix of strategies to see you through accumulated stress like Nancy Marble's. Here are 3 actions to take.

• Look ahead and plan—a good way to control stress that comes from a pileup of foreseeable demands.

• Talk matters through—especially useful for frequent arguments and misunderstandings.

• Seek expert consultation—helpful when you don't know how to cope but know you can't leave matters as they are.

Mrs. Marble realized that marital quarrels can be healthy or unhealthy. The healthy variety is a reasonable discussion of differences with an eye to working out the conflicts. Marital disputes that solve problems are worth the stress they cause. Marital disputes that serve only to vent angry feelings solve nothing, cause an increased level of angry arousal, and perpetuate the stress. Often a trained marriage counselor, social worker, or family therapist can provide important guidance to a couple in the turmoil of a life transition.

Mrs. Marble tried to get George to go with her to talk to a family therapist, but he refused, saying that the only problem was her temper. His denial angered Mrs. Marble even further, and this issue became a continuing stressor in their lives.

Healthy, satisfying sexual relations can be an important stress reducer, and, not surprisingly, strained or infrequent sexual relations can have the opposite effect. Nancy could have sought professional help to find ways to keep the problem from becoming chronic and a major source of stress.

Had Nancy realized the potential effects on her health of the combined stress of her sister's death and her husband's retirement, she might not have piled on further optional stressors. She might have handled the situation by giving fewer parties, by hiring some help for those she did give, by lowering her self-expectations and asking her guests to bring covered dishes, or by postponing her entertaining to a time when she had less to cope with. George Marble, feeling useless and at loose ends, might have enjoyed planning and doing some of the work for the parties had his wife only asked.

Nancy Marble's traffic violation was a typical outcome of being stressed. As we'll see, an increase in accidents is a common symptom of a stress overload. Once Nancy learned some of the stress management techniques outlined farther on, she had no further problems with driving too fast or not concentrating on the road.

Lastly, Mrs. Marble's final breakdown into tears wasn't a bad response despite her embarrassment. By allowing herself to cry, she actually let off steam and relaxed. Holding onto strong feelings can be exhausting and stressful, whereas releasing those feelings can be a great de-stressor.

Relief in tears

We should applaud some of the changes in society that have made it all right for men to cry. Many men, who haven't cried since childhood, are amazed at the relief it can bring when they're truly upset.

Plan the timing of important events

A useful adjunct to finding your score on the Holmes and Rahe scale is to make a chart of your next year and use it as a scheduling tool. First, make a list of all your ongoing stressors such as mortgages. Next, fill in such fixed dates as Christmas or school graduations. Although you obviously won't be able to plan for many major life changes, this chart can help you plan when to schedule such stressful events as in-law visits, vacations, and job changes so as not to overdraw your reserves of adaptation energy.

Remember: don't try to avoid changes, but do try to regulate the timing of those over which you have some control so that you can meet them head on with plenty of energy.

Daily hassles/daily uplifts

Does your life ever seem to be nothing but a series of little hassles, and do those hassles get you down?

"Sometimes between getting the baby her breakfast, riding that crowded train to work, then answering phones all day while I'm also trying to type letters, then getting home just in time to get to the crowded supermarket to buy dinner, I feel like I'm going to get an ulcer! I know all those things are just a part of life, but they really get me down. And I always seem to have some little cold. I mean it's not like my life is that hard. I know lots of people would look at my life and say I had it pretty easy. So why do I always feel so low and tired?"

A group of researchers at the University of California might have an answer for this distressed young

Hassles

Yes, researchers have compiled a hassles scale! Hassles are "the irritating, frustrating, distressing demands that to some degree characterize everyday transactions." You can use the top 10 hassles—they're on this page—to control stress.

parent. These researchers feel that the accumulated little *hassles* of day-to-day life can drive people into illness. With this in mind, these researchers recently devised the Hassles Scale. They define hassles as "the irritating, frustrating, distressing demands that to some degree characterize everyday transactions with the environment. They include annoying practical problems such as losing things or traffic jams, and fortuitous occurrences such as inclement weather as well as arguments, disappointments, and financial and family concerns."

These psychologists have identified 117 common daily hassles that most of the people they interviewed seemed to mention. Here are the top ten.

Hassles scale
1. Concerns about weight
2. Health of a family member
3. Rising prices of common goods
4. Home maintenance
5. Too many things to do
6. Misplacing or losing things
7. Yard work or outside home maintenance
8. Property, investment, or taxes
9. Crime
10. Physical appearance

How hassles affect you

Hassles might affect your health in several ways. They may simply accumulate until they become the straw that broke the camel's back. Hassles may also be the harmful ingredient in major life events. The death of a spouse or a divorce may be made all the more horrendous because suddenly you may be faced with single-handedly maintaining the house, the finances, the car, and the family. If you're not used to coping with the furnace, handling the bank accounts, dealing with the auto repair shop, or getting the children off to school, all these mundane details can add up to being as taxing as the major life event that brought them all on.

Some experts believe that what you think about

Simple de-stressors

1. Don't be ashamed to cry. Some people prefer to go out in the woods or to get into the shower so that they can cry in private.

2. Some people find that yelling helps relieve their tension. If you can't go off where no one will hear you, you can smother some of the noise by yelling into a pillow.

3. Hard exercise like running can work off a lot of stress, but make sure that you first do some warm-up exercises like gentle stretching of your arms and legs so that you don't pull any muscles.

4. Some people set up a punching bag or a tetherball just for the purpose of working off anger and tension instead of letting it build up in their bodies.

these little hassles determines whether or not they'll make you sick. For example, physical appearance may not be a hassle to all people, but it may be a real problem to someone who places great importance on looking good. Home maintenance might be an uplift to some divorced people who are glad to have total control of the home, but it might be a hassle for a divorced person who feels overwhelmed by the new and unfamiliar responsibility.

Daily uplifts

Life isn't all unpleasant surprises and irritations. Or at least it doesn't have to be. Daily hassles have a counterpart that the researchers at the University of California call *daily uplifts*. Daily uplifts may actually counteract the negative effects of daily hassles. The balance of hassles and uplifts may determine what effect day-to-day life has on your health.

Just as hassles and major life events may cause stress diseases, little daily uplifts may actually protect you against stress diseases—if you'll let them. These researchers are saying something different from what Holmes and Rahe said: according to these researchers,

You've the power
*Research in both humans
and animals is beginning to
show that our emotions and
attitudes can make a big
difference in our physical
health. There's more and
more scientific proof that
positive thinking really
does have power. So try to
see the good side of things,
and try to take pleasure in
some of the little things that
are right, even when other
things in your life seem to
be going wrong.*

good and bad life events aren't equally harmful. The little joys of life, like getting a good night's rest and enjoying nature, are important stress reducers. This way of thinking also leaves some room for personal responses. If you're the type of person who is "driven nuts" by irritating little things going wrong, you may be asking for health problems. On the other hand, if you can take the time out to appreciate some of the simple pleasures available to all of us—even in the middle of a divorce or other serious problem—your health may not suffer. And this may be the key reason why some people get sick when they're undergoing stress and why others stay well.

Here are the ten most frequently mentioned daily uplifts:

Daily uplifts
1. Relating well with your spouse or lover
2. Relating well with friends
3. Completing a task
4. Feeling healthy
5. Getting enough sleep
6. Eating out
7. Meeting your responsibilities
8. Visiting, phoning, or writing someone
9. Spending time with family
10. Home (inside) pleasing to you

Hardiness: beating Holmes and Rahe's odds

We all know people who have gone through a lot of major life changes and never been sick. If Dennis Santucci, whose wife and son were killed in a car accident right after he had lost his job, had taken the Holmes and Rahe quiz, he would have scored well over 300, yet he hasn't even had a cold for years. How could this be?

Some researchers have begun to ask themselves the same question. Why do some people remain in excellent health even while undergoing traumatic and taxing life events? These people may simply have better

Use your goals and values

Stress does lay some people low. How can you combine high stress and low sickness? The answer is: believe in yourself. If you know where you want to go, how you're to get there, and what prize is at the end of your journey, you'll have some control over what's happening—and that will help you thrive.

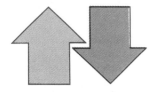

skills and resources for coping with life changes than do those who become ill. Or they are simply less bothered by things than other people are.

Suzanne C. Kobasa, a doctoral candidate at the University of Chicago, studied several hundred middle-aged male executives who had undergone enough life changes and demands for adaptation to run a high risk, according to Holmes and Rahe's scale. She divided her subjects into high stress/high illness and high stress/low illness categories and set out to find what made them tick and why their physiological responses to stress were different.

She found that the executives of the high stress/low illness group approached the necessary life changes with "a clear sense of (their) values, goals, and capabilities." Most important, she found, these men were strongly committed to themselves. "Staying healthy under stress," she writes, "is critically dependent upon a strong sense of commitment to self...an ability to recognize one's distinctive values, goals, and priorities." Instead of being passive, these people faced life and its changes with vigor.

Kobasa called this personality difference "hardiness." Hardy executives, she found, had a deep sense of meaningfulness. Instead of passively accepting life's changes, the hardy executives tried to see how such changes could be transformed into something beneficial to their overall life plan. Instead of feeling victimized by circumstances, no matter how bad, hardy individuals realize that they have some control over the outcome and take responsibility for making things work to their advantage.

Face stressors with hardiness

In addition to planning the timing of important life changes you can control, learn to face other stressors and daily hassles with hardiness:

• Believe that you can control or influence your situation. Feeling out of control is highly stressful. Even if you can't totally control the situation, chances are you

Attitude helps

What do pleasure and opportunity have in common? Both are good. "Sure," you may think, "but both are linked to success, and success is stressful." Try a change of attitude. Pleasure can be found, free and plentiful, if you'll slow down and let yourself see the gorgeous simplicity of a daisy, for example, or hear the surprising urgency of a cricket in late autumn. Opportunity is more than a chance to strike it rich. It's helping others, finding satisfaction in your work, making people laugh, soothing an upset child.

can gain a toehold in some small way. Maybe you can't quit that awful job right now, but maybe you can negotiate some changes with your supervisor. Maybe you can get more flexible hours, or take your breaks on a different schedule, or move away from the chatterbox at the next desk.

People who live successfully with alcoholic spouses learn that although they can't control the other person's drinking, they can control their own lives and reduce the pain of living in such a situation. "Just taking charge of myself and realizing that I could do something other than sitting there hoping I could change his ways changed the stress level of that time in our marriage." If you take responsibility for your own feelings and actions, the actions of other people have less power to hurt you and disrupt your life.

• Commit yourself to living life with pleasure, and enjoy its smallest details. In our rush to get ahead, to be successful, many of us forget to take pleasure in life itself. Listen to the birds sing, play with your child or your pets, talk to a friend. Enjoy life itself no matter what's going on. Try taking a few minutes out several times a day for just this purpose. Notice what's going on around you. No matter how serious your problems, a few minutes taken away from them aren't going to make them worse. And be sure to really leave your problems behind! So many people have the right idea to take time out for a walk or to daydream a little, but what do they do? They spend that time worrying about the same old problems. Think of this time as a few minutes to let fresh ideas come to your mind. You'll find that these periods aren't a waste of time. Rather, they'll give you energy and a better outlook for solving your problems when you return to them.

• Be committed to yourself. You don't have to be selfish about it, but remember your right to try to make your life meaningful to you. Only you can make your life mean what you want it to. Make a contract with yourself that you will take yourself and your goals seriously.

Better attitudes

Sometimes we make things harder on ourselves by concentrating on negative thoughts. "I'll never be able to do that," "I'm getting nowhere," "I can't cope." Change the way you talk to yourself. "I'm going to try my best to do that," "I may not be getting anywhere today, but look at everything I did yesterday," "I can take things in stride." These are better, more positive attitudes.

• Look at change as an opportunity to grow, to develop new potentials. Some people are terrified by change. They cling desperately to the comfortable assurances of their lives and so they grow very little. Such people cut themselves off from some of the greatest pleasures of life. Remember the old saying "nothing ventured, nothing gained"? Sometimes we have to risk change or at least allow it to happen. If we don't, we have no way of knowing what we're capable of, what life can give us.

Let change into your life in little ways. Change your routine. Take a different route to work, eat somewhere new, make a new friend. Change is energizing. You never know what new horizons you may be opening up!

• View crises and failures as learning experiences. See what they have to teach you and how you can use this new understanding. Nobody wants to fail, but we all do from time to time. You can learn just as much, if not more, from failure as you can from success. Instead of feeling embarrassed or not admitting your failures, examine them. Try to see what went wrong, whether you could have done something differently, and resolve to put your experience to use.

• Don't discount life's little joys and overemphasize its hassles. Lighten up! We live in a beautiful, mysterious world.

• Optimism and positive thinking are contagious. If you can smile through your days, you'll make other people smile along with you. Instead of creating a negative mood, you'll create a positive one. So smile, try to say something nice to other people even when you're feeling low. They'll return the favor.

3 Coping: the key to staying healthy

Who gets ulcers?
Are you surprised to hear that fewer bosses than workers get ulcers? Why? Bosses are in control and have the means to pass on some of their burdens. In contrast, many workers endure the stress without the control—a combination that can lead to sickness.

You've probably seen the Hollywood stereotype of the busy executive talking on two telephones at once, telling three secretaries what to do, and working long hours. These executives always seemed to have ulcers. This notion was based on research during the fifties showing that monkeys that had to expend a lot of energy turning off mild shocks ended up riddled with ulcers. The monkeys that sat back and did nothing, even if they received shocks they couldn't turn off, seemed to come out much better. Although they got some ulcers—probably from sitting there and being shocked—they were nowhere near as ill as the "executive monkeys" that were constantly having to "cope" with the shocks.

That model of executive stress hung on for a long time. In fact, although it has been disproved by thirty years of newer studies, many people still believe that top executives under pressure get ulcers and other stress diseases while the secretaries and messengers in their less influential jobs are much healthier.

Let's look at the results of a 1984 survey of 5,000 women conducted by *Working Woman* magazine. Their study noted that "Stress illnesses happen most to those who are under the greatest pressure but have the least influence....The top managers are healthiest." Just the opposite of those ulcer-prone executives. Time after time, studies of occupational health show that the bosses don't develop ulcers, insomnia, headaches, hypertension, heart diseases, and other disorders that we think of as stress diseases; but the people they're bossing do. Why? One group has control and the other doesn't.

The importance of control

The real importance of feeling in control was first demonstrated in studies during the early 1970s by Dr. Jay Weiss at Rockefeller University. His work contradicted the old stereotype of the executive who got sick because he was so busy being in control. In his studies, rats that could control their environment by turning off shocks suffered from fewer ulcers than the rats that couldn't do anything to control the shocks. Dr. Weiss's

How do you take control?

The first step toward control involves yourself. Review your responsibilities and chores. Decide on your priorities: what must you do first, second, and so on. Review your means: how can you do the first task—using what method and with whom? Determine what is not a priority and let it wait. Learning to say no to yourself and to others can help you get control over your responsibilities.

studies were confirmed with both humans and animals. Feeling helpless to change things you don't like is very stressful. A bad job, poor housing, an unhappy marriage do more damage to you if you feel that you have no alternative.

Coping and coping style are major determinants of how your health will fare when you're under stress. You can put this information to work by remembering that if you feel competent and able to cope, you're more resistant to various illnesses. None of us can be fully in control of every situation all the time, and we shouldn't try to be. Other people don't like having you control them, so don't try to. *Do try to be in control of yourself first of all and then of those things that are your responsibility.*

We feel out of control when we think we're being used. Try turning this feeling around. Your boss may be giving you a hard time and making you work overtime on projects that aren't even supposed to be part of your job. If you feel helpless and small, you're far more likely to become ill than if you think about how you can use your boss at the same time. Taking on extra projects may expand your skills so that you can go look for a better job elsewhere. If you consider your boss as a teacher, things can begin to look very different.

One writer said that he was never bothered too much by unpleasant, even tragic, experiences because he knew that they gave him things to write about. "I can turn any situation to my advantage in that way," he said. "To be a good writer, you have to have lived through things. Although unpleasant things make me unhappy, a little voice inside tells me I should be thankful that I have lived firsthand through another experience that could later enrich my work."

Even if you're not a writer, you can use many of the less happy things that happen to you as learning experiences. You can help control how bad things will affect you by telling yourself that you'll learn from whatever comes your way and that you'll turn bad things into something good later on. Amazingly, telling yourself to look for the positive core in bad experiences robs them of their power to hurt you.

Environmental stressors

We've seen how life events and the day-to-day hassles of living may cause stress, but before we leave this discussion of the common stressors in our lives, we should explore *environmental* stressors.

Stress control chart

You can take control of your responsibilities and chores by constructing a chart of them. Write down the tasks you have to do (in the order of their importance), the means you have to accomplish the tasks, and the factors you'll need to remember to perform the tasks successfully.

Here's an example of a stress control chart in action—in this case, a busy executive reviewing last-minute preparations for a vacation. Follow the steps outlined here to prepare your own stress control chart, suited to your needs.

Tasks in order of importance	Means to accomplish the tasks	Factors to remember
1. Complete monthly report	Schedule update from Earl; reserve computer time	Earl's out of town next 3 days; computer program needs update
2. Confirm reservations	Have travel agent confirm all dates	Bob's hours are 2–8 p.m.
3. Reserve kennel time	Call Eleanor and mail check	Requires two weeks' notice
4. Interrupt mail and other deliveries	Go to post office; call delivery services	Ask Rosalie to double-check for first 3 or 4 days
5. Confirm Rosalie on home checks	Have Sophie make a dinner reservation	Remind Rosalie of the key's location and how to shut off the alarm

Unless you live in an idyllic country setting, you're probably experiencing a certain amount of stress just from your surroundings. Noise, crowding, crime, pollution are all potential stressors that your body may be adapting to day in and day out.

You may be adapting successfully to your surroundings, but what toll are these constant adaptations going to take on your health? People who live near an airport eventually begin not to hear the noise, but researchers still find that they suffer from an increased incidence of certain types of illnesses.

Some of the most informative research on environmental stress was done by Drs. Jerome E. Singer and David C. Glass, who often used noise as the stressor in their experiments. Singer and Glass found that al-

Analyze your environment

Do a stress analysis of your environment. First list those elements that bother you — noise, glare, stuffy air, whatever (the picture on page 29 may give you other suggestions). Then list one or more changes that you might make to neutralize each stressor. List an action even if you're not sure you can yet bring it about. It'll give you food for thought.

though people do adapt to just about any environmental stressor, such adaptation eventually takes its toll. Many environmental stressors are all the more dangerous because they occur well below the level that would cause actual physical damage. Their effects are subtle and indirect. Singer and Glass say that workers from noisy offices are less efficient, less polite, and less able to tolerate frustration than those from a more tranquil work environment. Of course, some loud noise at close range, such as that from subways and jackhammers, packs the double whammy of causing both hearing damage as well as these same subtle effects on behavior and health.

Over the course of their studies, Singer and Glass found three factors that can lessen the damage resulting from environmental stressors:

- Predictability
- Social context
- Feeling of control.

Predictability greatly lessens the effects of a stressor. Once you've gotten used to something and know it's going to happen, even if it's unpleasant, your body acts with a far smaller degree of alarm. For instance, if you live on a railroad line where trains run by on schedule, your body will eventually get used to the sounds and react less than if you live on a major road where 18 wheelers rumble by at odd and unpredictable hours. Glass and Singer found that unpredictable noise also caused more disrupted after-noise behavior in human subjects.

The *context* in which something occurs is important in determining its effects on your health. If you enjoy people around you at all times, you may find it jolly— not stressful at all—to live in a noisy apartment building. If, on the other hand, you grew up in a rural environment and need plenty of personal space, the noise in such a building might be very upsetting to you.

We have already examined experimental evidence that clearly shows that having a sense of *control* reduces stress, while a sense of being helpless to control or influence your environment increases the likelihood that you'll become ill. Drs. Singer and Glass illustrate this theory by citing a Swedish study of commuters. Those who got on at the beginning of the line experienced less stress than those who got on later and rode only half as long to get to work. The rea-

Reducing environmental stressors

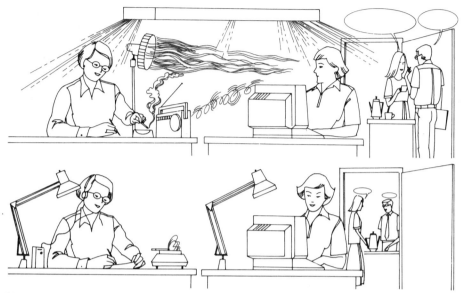

Glare from lights, noise from a radio and nearby people on a break, drifting smoke, and a misdirected fan make office life stressful for the person on the right in the top picture. After a few changes, the stressors are gone: soft lights, radio earphones, coffee maker in the hall, a smoke filter machine, and the fan removed.

son? Those who got on at the beginning had total control over where they sat, whom they sat with, and how they arranged their packages and briefcases. Those who got on later had to take whatever seats they could get and therefore were unable to structure their environment as they wished.

Since we can't always flee our environment or fight it, we need to learn ways of dealing with environmental stress.

Handling environmental stress

Try to arrange your environment so that it's less stressful. At one end of the spectrum is actually escaping it by moving elsewhere. However, ear plugs, insulation, a white noise generator, or a radio playing music you like are some ways you can control noise. Rearranging desks at work may help reduce a noise or privacy problem. Changing your schedule slightly might solve your problem with rush hour traffic.

Convincing yourself that something you find stressful is actually necessary may place it in a more favorable context and lessen the toll it exacts. The noise and dirt of the big city may bother you a lot less if, for instance, you can convince yourself that these are part of the excitement of being in the center of things where you have a chance to be recognized in your work.

Feeling a sense of control is all-important in reducing the physical effects of environmental stressors.

Some "relaxants" actually add to stress: smoking, drugs, alcohol. Find other ways to relax, such as exercise, biofeedback, or meditation.

One secretary recalled how much less frustration she felt with her chain-smoking co-worker when she took matters into her own hands and bought a desktop air cleaner. Now she's no longer bothered that she can't convince the smoker to stop.

Finally, when you can't control your environment enough to make a difference, you can learn to react less to stressors. Stress management techniques can help you let stressors roll off your back.

Stressful coping styles

In their attempt to cope with stressful lives, many people develop unhealthy behaviors such as smoking, drug-taking, and drinking that may seem to help but actually are significant biological stressors in their own right.

Smoking

By now, almost all of us know that cigarette smoking is an extremely dangerous habit with nothing to recommend it. Perhaps 90 percent of all lung cancer could be avoided if people didn't smoke. In the next year or two, lung cancer will surpass breast cancer as the leading cause of cancer death among women. Not only are cigarettes implicated in lung disease, they are also factors in cancers of the stomach, mouth, tongue, esophagus, and bladder. Smokers also have more ulcers. And perhaps because smoking increases the amount of cholesterol in the blood, it's a major contributor to cardiovascular diseases. Yet people still smoke—many of them in a misguided attempt to cope with the anxiety and tension that fill their bodies; many of them because they're addicted.

The addictive ingredient in tobacco is nicotine. Because nicotine causes adrenalin release, each cigarette basically triggers a small fight or flight response that raises your blood pressure and makes your heart work harder. As a by-product of burning, cigarettes fill your blood with carbon monoxide, the same deadly gas that is found in auto exhaust. Carbon monoxide is taken up by the body in preference to oxygen, so that smokers often have blood carbon monoxide levels that are many times higher than those of nonsmokers. Carbon monoxide prevents sufficient oxygen from reaching the brain and other organs. Small doses cause severe headaches, mental dullness, dizziness, and irritability. Large doses in a confined space are commonly used as a means of suicide.

One of the most significant body chemical discov-

Carbon monoxide

Carbon monoxide is produced wherever something is burned. Common sources of carbon monoxide in our environment are cigarettes, auto exhaust, and heaters such as kerosene heaters and wood stoves. Unvented kerosene heaters are particularly dangerous because their toxic gases stay indoors. The major part of a wood stove's carbon monoxide goes up the chimney and doesn't enter your room.

Even though we require oxygen for life, for some curious reason our bodies will choose poisonous carbon monoxide over life-sustaining oxygen. When we inhale this invisible, odorless gas, it behaves like oxygen by combining with hemoglobin, a protein in our blood that normally transports oxygen throughout the body. Poisonous carbon monoxide, which is not usable by the body, is then delivered to the cells in place of oxygen.

The body's unexplained preference for carbon monoxide doesn't usually pose a problem unless we're breathing it in a confined space where fresh air is at a minimum. This may happen if you're using a kerosene heater in a small space without ventilation or if you're chain smoking. In these cases, you may develop extremely high levels of carbon monoxide in your blood. Breathing too much carbon monoxide can eventually kill you if you don't get some fresh air. Early signs of a carbon monoxide overload are dizziness, headache, nausea, and a flushed complexion. If you find this happening to you, get outdoors or to a source of fresh air. If you must use a kerosene heater, follow the manufacturer's instructions exactly, and make certain you have adequate ventilation.

eries has been a class of protein known as *endorphins*. These substances are chemically similar to opiates such as morphine and other painkillers except that they occur naturally in your body. Endorphins are released in response both to pain and to certain stressors. When your endorphin levels increase, you feel more pain-free, relaxed, and euphoric.

Cigarette smoking causes endorphin release, and this may be one reason why some people find the habit so hard to break. Just as opiates are addictive, some researchers now feel that we may become "addicted" to our own endorphins. Since each time you light a cigarette you are getting a dose of soothing endorphins, you tend to want to keep on having cigarettes. Accordingly, some behavioral scientists now feel that giving up smoking is easier if you substitute some other habit that causes the release of endorphins. Hard aerobic exercise seems to do this. Therefore, some people may find an exercise program an excellent adjunct to a smoke-ending program.

Marijuana

Less is known about marijuana than about tobacco. Because marijuana smoke is hotter, and is held deep in the lungs for a longer time, chronic use almost certainly causes severe lung and heart damage. Marijuana is also stored in fatty tissues throughout the body. No one yet knows the effects of chronic high-level marijuana usage. Until more is known, pregnant women and individuals with known lung or heart disease should stay away from it.

Alcohol

When used in moderation, alcohol can be a legitimate stress reducer. What is moderation? Most doctors now agree that up to two ounces of alcohol a day can actually help us unwind. Drinking at this moderate level is associated with greater longevity than either extreme of teetotaling or alcohol abuse. Small amounts of alcohol also seem to increase the ratio of HDL-C (high-density lipoprotein cholesterol) to LDL-C (low-density lipoprotein cholesterol). This is beneficial, because HDL appears to protect against coronary heart disease, while LDL appears to increase the risk of it.

Drinking more than two ounces of alcohol each day causes real problems when substituted for healthier coping mechanisms:

• Alcohol consumption, like the vigilance response, causes your adrenals to release cortisol, a stress hormone that can raise blood pressure by causing your kidneys to retain salt.

Comparing alcohol content by volume

The percentage of alcohol varies according to the kind of drink. An ounce of beer has less alcohol than an ounce of whiskey, but if you drink three or four beers, you come near drinking the same amount of alcohol contained in an ounce of whiskey. Many people avoid the problems of alcohol by learning to enjoy nonalcoholic beverages, like decaffeinated iced tea or coffee, sparkling water, or an occasional low-calorie or low-alcohol beer.

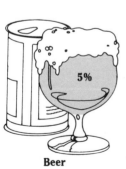

Beer 5%

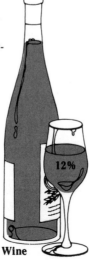

Wine 12%

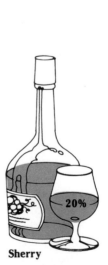

Sherry 20%

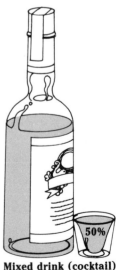

Mixed drink (cocktail) 50%

Caffeine

In our harried world, we're always having to do things faster and faster. Yet stress often makes us feel exhaused and drained of the energy needed to do things faster or even on time. Millions upon millions of us then turn to a stimulant for help. That stimulant is caffeine, and you can find it in your cup of tea or coffee and in soft drinks. Some people even go so far as to buy it in concentrated form in over-the-counter pep pills.

More doctors are now advising their patients to limit their caffeine intake, because like other stimulants caffeine causes many of the same changes in your body that stress does. If you're already in a state of alarm and then drink several cups of coffee, you'll have a lot of stimulants whizzing around in your body, hopping you up and making you feel tense.

Three or fewer caffeine beverages each day are enough. If you're drinking more than this, cut down. You may not feel so great for the first few days of cutting down. Caffeine is mildly addictive, so you may have headaches and feel tired and unable to concentrate at first. These feelings will disappear.

• Alcohol has a direct toxic effect on heart muscle and on other muscles because it depresses the nervous system. Thiamine (Vitamin B1) deficiency that often accompanies alcohol abuse may also damage the heart, making it pump less efficiently.

• Alcohol abuse may cause irreversible liver damage, both as a direct effect and as a result of the poor diet of many alcohol abusers.

Of the millions of problem drinkers in the United States, many began overdrinking as a misguided attempt at dealing with the stresses of life. Yet alcohol abuse does nothing to relieve stress. In fact, it increases requirements for your body's precious store of adaptation energy and, in the long run, shortens your life.

Behavioral and chemical treatments for alcohol abuse depend upon the individual drinker. Your family physician or the chemical dependency unit of a nearby hospital should be the first stop when you're trying to control this habit. Alcoholics Anonymous (AA) has had enormous success in helping former drinkers. All major cities have several AA groups, and most communities have at least one chapter.

Tranquilizers

Valium is one of the most widely prescribed brand name drugs in the United States. Millions of people are taking it and other tranquilizers in an attempt to soothe tension and anxiety. Even harder on the body are the barbiturates, which depress your central nervous system and act more to anesthetize than to relax you. Barbiturates are highly addictive, and abrupt withdrawal from them is potentially life-threatening and should only be undertaken in a hospital. While doctors used to believe that Valium and related drugs such as Dalmane were relatively safe and nonaddictive, we now know that these drugs too can be abused.

None of the behaviors we've just discussed is a useful way of coping with stress, because each only adds to the body's stress level and doesn't give you a sense of influence or control over your environment—at least not for very long. On top of being ineffectual for coping with stress, these behaviors are actually harmful and may contribute to the development of some of the diseases of adaptation discussed in the next chapter.

4

Stress diseases

What is blood pressure?

Your blood carries oxygen and other nutrients as well as hormones to all your body's cells. Your blood pressure is simply the measurement of the pressure your circulating blood exerts on the walls of your blood vessels. In order to circulate through the miles of blood vessels throughout your body, your blood must be under pressure.

Anything that your body or mind has to adjust to causes some degree of stress response. If the stress continues and you adapt and begin to cope effectively, the stress response is turned off. If, however, the stress response is kept up over long periods, eventually some system in your body breaks down, and your overall health suffers in some way.

The breakdown often occurs in some part of your body that is already weak. For instance, you may have inherited a weak heart (even though it has never given you any trouble). Forty years of overreactions to stress plus a faulty diet may finally cause you to develop heart disease.

As we've seen, stress may also lead you to try coping behaviors such as smoking and drinking that cause illness in and of themselves. The sad example of the person who tries to control his tension by smoking two packs of cigarettes a day and then develops cancer is an all too familiar example of this indirect effect of stress on disease.

Stress and your reactions to stress can cause or worsen diseases like hypertension, heart disease, cancer, asthma, and ulcers, and the disorders like headaches, dental problems, and back problems.

Hypertension

Jack Riley had been seeing his family doctor fairly frequently over the past year. His doctor had wanted Jack to keep an eye on his blood pressure, which was a bit higher than the desirable range. His doctor had recommended that Jack cut back on salt, stop smoking, and exercise regularly. Jack did his best to follow these instructions, although he did occasionally lose his resolve and smoke a few cigarettes.

His doctor took a blood pressure reading, but instead of putting his blood pressure gauge away, he kept it out. After examining Jack's eyes, he took another reading. "It's still high, Jack. It's 155/95, and I really feel that it's time to start you on some medication."

"But, doc," protested Jack. "I can't be sick. I feel great, I never miss work, I don't have any problems, I don't drink or smoke…"

Some doctors call it the "Silent Killer." Hyperten-

The circulatory system

The largest blood vessels are the arteries, which carry red, oxygen-enriched blood from your heart and lungs. Arteries divide into smaller and smaller units in order to reach every part of your body. Like a main highway, the arteries feed into arterioles or smaller roads that in turn feed into the small roads known as capillaries. The blood is returned to the heart and lungs through larger and larger veins. Other wastes are carried to the kidneys, where they are excreted in the urine. While the arteries have muscular walls and can expand somewhat under increased pressure, the veins can't.

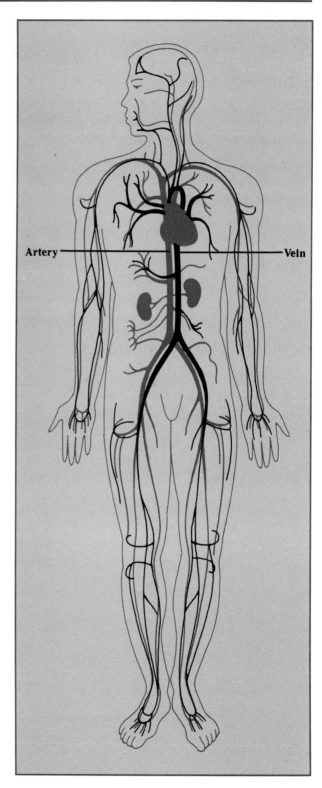

Artery ⸺⸺⸺⸺⸺⸺⸺⸺ Vein

sion, or high blood pressure, is one of America's major diseases. Possibly one in three adult Americans has hypertension, and another 25 million have borderline hypertension that fluctuates from the normal into the abnormal range. Amazingly, many people with severe hypertension don't even know they have it for, despite its name, it has nothing to do with extreme tension. You can lead a relaxed, tranquil life and still have dangerously high blood pressure without any visible sign of it.

A puzzling statistic
Hypertension is nearly twice as common among blacks as in the rest of the population. In fact, some 30 percent of black adults have hypertension. No one knows why.

While stress often plays a role in hypertension, it isn't the cause. As we'll see, hypertension can be caused by genetic, physiological, or dietary factors or any combination of these. Hypertension is easy, inexpensive, and painless to detect. If caught early, it's usually fairly easy to control with medication and dietary modification. However, if left alone, it's highly damaging and will cut years off your life.

The blood pressure reading

Blood pressure is recorded as two numbers, and when your doctor or nurse takes your blood pressure, he or she should tell you the values of the numbers. The top number represents your systolic pressure, the pressure in your arteries when your heart is in its pumping phase. If you put your fingers at one of the pulse points at your wrists or along the side of your neck, you'll feel the rhythm of your beating heart. You'll notice a split second of inactivity between beats. This relaxed phase is called the diastole. The lower blood pressure number represents this diastolic, or resting, pressure.

Your doctor or nurse measures your blood pressure by wrapping the pressure-sensitive cuff of a device known as a sphygmomanometer around your arm. He or she then inflates the cuff, which presses on the main artery in your arm, until the blood flow is cut off. Your doctor or nurse then listens through a stethoscope for your heart's pumping and resting sounds and watches the column of mercury (or the needle in a gauge) on the sphygmomanometer fall to arrive at your blood pressure reading.

While a reading of 120/80 is sometimes considered average and normal for adults, the upper number (systolic pressure) may range 20 points in either direction (for example, from 100 to 140). The lower number (diastolic pressure) may range ten points (for example, from 80 to 90). A pressure of 140/90 is considered mild hypertension.

Measuring blood pressure

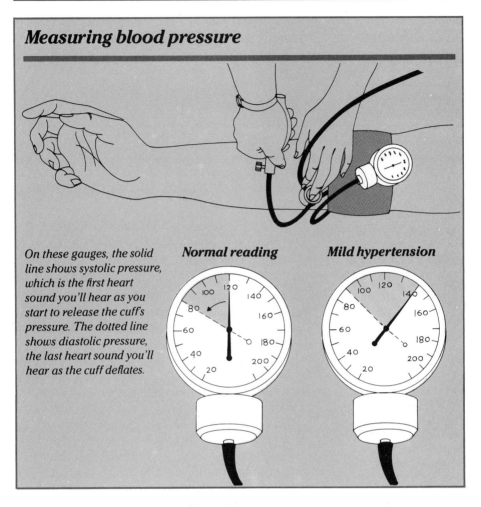

On these gauges, the solid line shows systolic pressure, which is the first heart sound you'll hear as you start to release the cuff's pressure. The dotted line shows diastolic pressure, the last heart sound you'll hear as the cuff deflates.

Normal reading

Mild hypertension

Blood pressure and hypertension

Hypertension means that your heart is having to work too hard to pump blood through your body to nourish your tissues.

Your blood pressure may rise because your heart is putting out an increased amount of blood with each pump. This happens commonly when a salt overload causes you to retain excess fluids and you have more blood for your heart to pump. Or the muscular walls of the arterial system may constrict, forcing the blood through a smaller opening, which drives up the pressure. Another common cause of hypertension is blockage of the arteries by fatty debris that clings to the arterial walls and narrows the opening that the blood must pass through. This condition forces the blood pressure to increase. In the worst case, all of these processes may be taking place.

Stress and hypertension: new clues

A recent study by Kathleen Light, MD, and her colleagues at the North Carolina School of Medicine has provided evidence to explain how stress can cause hypertension in susceptible individuals.

Young male volunteers were divided into high and low hypertension risk groups. The high risk group had either borderline hypertension or one or two hypertensive parents. The low risk group had no personal or family history of the disease. When the high risk men had to play a difficult video game and compete with a partner in doing so, their bodies responded very differently from those of the low risk volunteers. They showed a greatly increased heart rate in response to the challenge, and they retained higher quantities of salt and fluids, which, as we have seen, can raise blood pressure. Some of the low risk subjects also showed an increased heart rate, but not the accompanying changes in salt and fluid retention.

Causes and treatment of hypertension

Much research has gone into the causes and treatment of essential hypertension, and doctors now have some clues.

Heredity. Many hypertensives have the disease in their family. If one of your parents had or has the disease, the chance you or one of your siblings will develop the disease is fifty-fifty. If both your parents had it, your risk is 90 percent. Many researchers suspect that a family may pass along some undetectably small kidney defect that causes the body to keep raising its own blood pressure.

Smoking. Smoking has nothing to recommend it. Hypertension is another of the diseases that can be worsened by smoking.

Diet. If you have hypertension, your doctor may advise you to cut back on salt (sodium). That's because a lot of evidence suggests that too much salt can worsen hypertension by causing you to retain fluids and increasing your circulation volume.

Salt is essential for life. Among its functions in the body are regulation of fluid balance, the electrical stimulation of heart muscle, and the transmission of nerve impulses. The most common source of salt in our diets is sodium chloride, or common table salt, but we may also take in substantial quantities in other forms. Monosodium glutamate, sodium nitrite, and sodium benzoate are but a few of the sodium compounds that we may eat every day. They're used as taste enhancers and preservatives in a variety of foods ranging from pudding mix to cold cuts, soda, and many Oriental dishes.

Most of us eat many times more salt than we need. Our bodies require only about one to one-and-a-half teaspoons daily from any source in order to function optimally. This means that you really don't have to add any salt to your food. As long as you're eating meat, dairy products, or bread, chances are you're getting plenty of salt. If you eat processed foods to any extent, chances are you're overloading.

Many researchers now believe that salt overload is a major factor in over half the cases of essential hypertension. While the normal healthy kidney can eliminate all the salt you eat, not all of us are born with that perfectly functioning kidney. That salt-sensitive 60 percent of essential hypertensives may be those whose kidneys, for one reason or another, can't handle excess salt.

How salt affects blood pressure

Many of us liberally add salt to our food without giving it a second thought. But for someone with hypertension, this commonly used seasoning is a luxury that should be used sparingly. Here's why.

Nearly half of salt is comprised of sodium, the mineral that causes fluid retention in the body. Fluid retention tends to increase blood volume, which raises peripheral resistance and boosts blood pressure.

By gradually decreasing salt consumption, you help reduce blood volume and peripheral resistance. When arterial blood flow encounters less resistance, blood pressure drops.

Nonprescription drugs that contain salt

Product	Salt content
Alka-Seltzer	551 mg/tablet
Alka-Seltzer Plus Cold Medicine	515 mg/tablet
Bisodol	157 mg/tsp
Cerose-DM	39 mg/ml of sodium citrate
Correctol	7.82 mg/tablet
Di-Gel	8.5 mg/tsp
Maalox Plus	1.38 mg/tsp
Metamucil	10 mg/tbs
Rolaids	53 mg/tablet
Soda Mint Tablets	88.7 mg/tablet
Tussar-2	26 mg/ml of sodium citrate
Vicks Formula 44 Cough Mixture	50 mg/ml of sodium citrate

Nonprescription drugs that don't contain salt

- Bayer
- Bufferin
- CoTylenol
- Comtrex
- Contac
- Coricidin
- Ecotrin
- Excedrin
- Midol
- Nytol
- Pamprin
- Pepto-Bismol
- Phillips' Milk of Magnesia
- Robitussin-DM
- Sine-Aid
- Sine-Off
- Sominex
- Sudafed
- Triaminic Syrup
- Triaminic Expectorant
- Traminicin
- Tylenol
- Vanquish

Other causes. Obesity may also cause hypertension. In a small percentage of women, oral contraceptives will cause a rise in blood pressure that almost always reverses when the pills are discontinued.

Stress and hypertension are related in several ways. If continually triggered, the stress response may lead to hypertension even in those who don't eat too much salt, whose families have been free of the disease for generations, and who exercise daily and maintain a trim waistline. In those who already have hypertension, the additional factor of too much stress can be a deadly combination.

(Text continues on page 42.)

Cutting down on sodium

To help control high blood pressure, avoid as many salty foods as you can. Include more low-sodium foods and get out of the habit of adding salt to your food.

Read what follows for some practical advice. Then, review this chart for details on low-sodium foods to enjoy and high-sodium foods to avoid.

• Season foods with herbs and spices.

• Use fresh tomatoes whenever possible for soups and sauces, or use unsalted canned tomatoes, tomato paste, or unsalted tomato juice.

• Season vegetables with vegetable oil, margarine, or spices like parsley or sweet basil.

• Rinse canned foods (including vegetables, tuna, and cottage cheese) under running water to reduce the sodium content.

• Read product labels carefully, keeping in mind that additives are listed in order of greatest quantity. Avoid a product if one of these additives is among the first five listed: salt, sodium benzoate, sodium nitrate, or monosodium glutamate (MSG).

• At restaurants, order boiled, baked, broiled, or roasted foods. Skip gravies, juices, soups, and cheesy dressings.

• Avoid salt substitutes and light salt, unless your doctor approves.

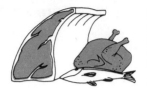

Meat
Low-sodium foods:
Poultry, fresh or frozen fish, veal, lamb, pork, beef
High-sodium foods:
Sausage, hot dogs, ham, bacon, luncheon meats, salt pork, smoked fish, herring, sardines, canned meat, TV dinners

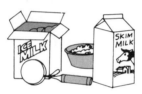

Dairy products
Low-sodium foods:
Skim milk, low-fat cottage cheese, ice milk
High-sodium foods:
Cheese (especially processed), buttermilk, ice cream

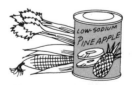

Fruits and vegetables
Low-sodium foods:
All fresh, frozen, and low-sodium canned fruits and vegetables
High-sodium foods:
Olives, pickles, sauerkraut, canned vegetables

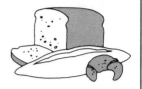

Breads and cereals
Low-sodium foods:
Most commercial and homemade breads
High-sodium foods:
Salted crackers, pretzels, rye rolls

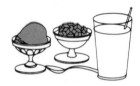

Snack foods
Low-sodium foods:
Sherbet, fruit ice, gelatin, fruit drinks
High-sodium foods:
Potato chips, pork rind, salted nuts, salted popcorn

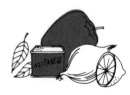

Seasonings
Low-sodium foods:
Fresh garlic, fresh onion, bay leaf, pepper, dill, nutmeg, rosemary, green pepper, lemon juice.
High-sodium foods:
Salt, garlic or onion salt, bouillon, soy sauce, meat tenderizers, canned soups

Guide to potassium-rich foods

Your doctor may have prescribed a water pill (diuretic) to help control your blood pressure. Because this medication may result in the loss of an electrolyte (chemical) called potassium, he or she may ask you to eat more potassium-rich foods.

The numbers listed below indicate the amount of potassium (in milligrams) found in 100 grams (3½-ounce serving) of food. All of these foods are high in potassium—but some of them are high in calories, too. So if you're on a low calorie diet, check with your doctor for further guidelines.

Too little potassium can cause muscle cramps (especially in the legs), muscle weakness, paralysis, and spasms. If you still have these problems after adding potassium to your diet, call your doctor.

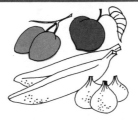

Fruits	mg
Apricots	281
Bananas	370
Dates	648
Figs	152
Nectarines	294
Oranges	200
Peaches	202
Plums	299
Prunes	262
Raisins	355

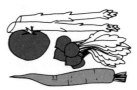

Vegetables	mg
Asparagus	238
Brussels sprouts	295
Cabbage	233
Carrots	341
Endive	294
Lima beans	394
Peppers	213
Potatoes	407
Radishes	322
Spinach	324
Sweet potatoes	300

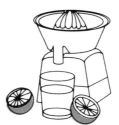

Juices	mg
Orange, fresh or	200
reconstituted	186
Tomato	227

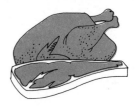

Meats	mg
Beef	370
Chicken	411
Lamb	290
Liver	380
Pork	326
Turkey	411
Veal	500

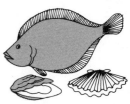

Fish	mg
Bass	256
Flounder	342
Haddock	348
Halibut	525
Oysters	203
Perch	284
Salmon	421
Sardines, canned	590
Scallops	476
Tuna	301

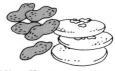

Miscellaneous	mg
Gingersnap cookies	462
Graham crackers	384
Oatmeal cookies (with raisins)	370
Ice milk	195
Milk, dry (nonfat solids)	1,745
Molasses (light)	917
Peanuts	674
Peanut butter	670

Are you a hot reactor?

Finding out whether you're a hot reactor involves taking your blood pressure reading while you're at rest and again after you've performed several standard tests. In his book *Is It Worth Dying For?*, Dr. Robert S. Eliot suggests several tests. One involves plunging your hand into a bucket or basin of ice water for 70 seconds. Playing a video game or making yourself do difficult mental arithmetic are also tests that you can use. Also test yourself after going through a typical daily hassle such as asking your children to clean up their rooms or having an argument with your boss. Take your reading immediately after the stress or the test that you choose. Dr. Eliot also cautions that you must do the testing over several weeks and average out your blood pressure readings.

Perhaps you can arrange to have your doctor do this testing on you. You can also do the testing at home if you have blood pressure equipment and know how to use it. The new electronic type, although twice as expensive as the mercury column and stethoscope method, is far easier for the inexperienced person to use.

If you find that either part of your average blood pressure rises to the 140/90 range while testing, you need to see a doctor. If your resting blood pressure is normal, you will not need anti-hypertensive medication. The most effective way of dealing with hot reacting in the face of a normal resting blood pressure is to learn to use some of the stress management techniques presented farther on.

To be sure

If you test your blood pressure at home and find that it's high, don't worry. Sometimes when you're feeling nervous or stressed, your blood pressure rises temporarily. Don't assume that you have hypertension on the basis of one blood pressure reading. Take a couple of readings when you're feeling calm and relaxed. If your blood pressure reading is still high after a couple of readings on different days, see your doctor.

Hot reactors

Some people who may appear as cool as cucumbers are actually boiling inside. When these people find themselves in a stressful situation, their blood pressure soars without their even knowing it. Dr. Robert Eliot, director of the National Center of Preventive and Stress Medicine, has coined the name "hot reactors" for such people.

In one experiment conducted by Dr. Eliot and his colleagues in their stress lab, healthy male volunteers between the ages of 25 and 65 were asked to do quick mental calculations or to play a challenging video game. The results were surprising and frightening: 17 percent of these healthy men reacted to these fairly minor challenges with sudden blood pressure increases up to the dangerous level of 160/95, definitely hypertensive.

Hot reacting is a massively overzealous alarm reaction to a stressor of little real consequence. While many of us overract to minor stressors, not all of us develop high blood pressure while so doing. Hot reactors release large quantities of stress hormones that cause an inappropriate cardiovascular response and temporary hypertension.

Some researchers feel that such repeated overreactions to stress and the reversible rises in blood pressure that accompany them can eventually cause permanent hypertension. This may happen because the body gets used to the higher pressure that may occur many times each day and finally "resets" itself so that the higher pressure is perceived as normal.

Hot reacting is particularly dangerous because those who have this problem have absolutely no idea that their bodies are making this inappropriate response.

The dangers of hypertension

Hypertension is dangerous for several reasons. Not only is it a serious disease in its own right, but it's also a major risk factor for heart disease, strokes, and kidney disease. If left untreated, essential hypertension will eventually turn into the more serious condi-

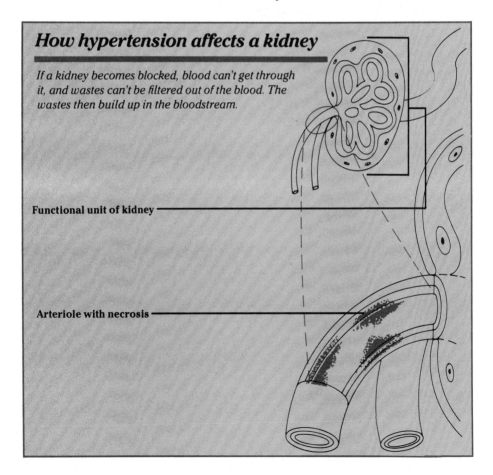

How hypertension affects a kidney

If a kidney becomes blocked, blood can't get through it, and wastes can't be filtered out of the blood. The wastes then build up in the bloodstream.

Functional unit of kidney

Arteriole with necrosis

Exercise and hypertension

Exercise is very important in the management of hypertension. Nobody is sure why exercise is so helpful, but many studies show that people's blood pressure (and cholesterol) lowers with exercise. In some cases, an exercise program alone will be enough to control a mild case of hypertension. If you do start an exercise program, be sure to talk to your doctor first and to start slowly so that you don't cause any problems.

tion known as malignant hypertension. This means that vital organs have become involved. The most common complications involve the blood vessels of the retina, the part of your eye that "sees." The heart, the kidneys, and the blood vessels of the brain are other common sites of organ damage caused by severe hypertension.

People with hypertension may be totally symptom-free, although some people may experience headaches, dizziness, or tingling in the limbs. Since these symptoms don't seem very dangerous, people usually try to treat them with aspirin and other easily available remedies. The first news you have of the disease may be at your next physical. For this reason, have your blood pressure checked at least annually. Even if you don't have a full physical, most doctors are happy to let you stop by for a blood pressure check. Health fairs and community health services usually offer free

High blood pressure drugs and sex

The drugs used to counteract hypertension may interfere with a patient's sex life. If you develop sex problems while you're taking an antihypertensive, tell your doctor. A change of drug may solve your problem.

The following chart matches some of these drugs to their possible adverse effects.

Drug	Adverse effect
Atenolol *(Tenormin)*	impotence
Chlorthialidone *(Hygroton)*	decreased sexual drive; impotence
Guanethidine *(Ismelin)*	impotence; no ejaculation
Hydralazine *(Apresoline* and others*)*	impotence
Methyldopa *(Aldomet)*	decreased sexual drive; impotence; delayed or no ejaculation
Phenoxybenzamine *(Dibenzyline)*	no ejaculation
Prazosin *(Minipress)*	impotence
Propranolol *(Inderal)*	loss of sexual drive; impotence
Reserpine	decreased sexual drive; impotence; decreased or no ejaculation
Spironolactone *(Aldactone)*	decreased sexual drive; impotence
Thiazide diuretics	impotence
Timolol *(Blocadren, Timolide)*	decreased sexual drive; impotence

blood pressure monitoring, but you can't rely on a single reading. If you use these services, have the test done several times on different days.

Patients with untreated essential hypertension have a life expectancy of about twenty years after the onset of the disease. The disease may stay in a fairly benign phase for as long as fifteen years if left untreated, but eventually major organ damage begins.

The good news is that hypertension, particularly when caught early, can be treated. Most cases of hypertension can't be cured, but medication can keep the disease under control. Sometimes, borderline hypertension can be normalized by following a low-salt diet, losing weight, exercising, and using meditation or other relaxation techniques.

Your doctor may prescribe any of several types of anti-hypertensive medications alone or in combination.

• Diuretics can help lower blood pressure by decreasing the amount of fluid your kidneys retain.

• Beta blockers work to control blood pressure by blocking the effects of the stress hormones epinephrine and norepinephrine and reducing the pumping rate of the heart.

• Vasodilators can reduce blood pressure by enlarging (dilating) the walls of the arteries so that the blood flows against less resistance.

If you have hypertension, you should take whatever medication your doctor prescribes and follow your doctor's orders. This may not be easy: some of these medications have bad side effects that make people dislike taking them. (If you have side effects with one medicine, you may not have them if your doctor changes you to another medicine.) However, failure to take medication will cause the disease to progress, with increasing damage to your body. Effective blood pressure control will add years to your life, even if you have already had some organ damage.

Heart disease

Your heart is a muscle that's constantly in motion from the day you're born to the day you die. If you consider how tired the muscles of your legs become after only an hour or so of running, you can appreciate what a truly extraordinary piece of machinery your heart is.

Your heart's job is to pump blood to every part of your body. Your heart works by contracting to squeeze

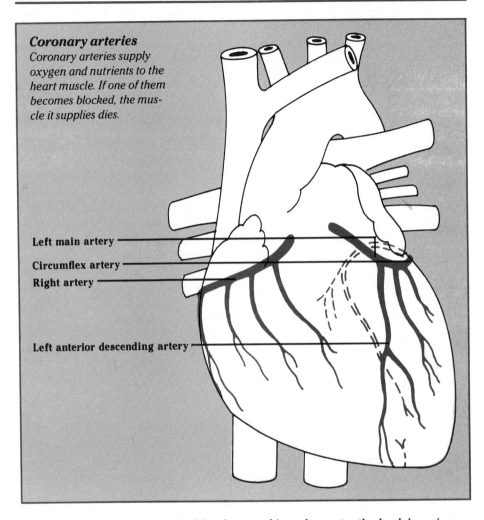

Coronary arteries

Coronary arteries supply oxygen and nutrients to the heart muscle. If one of them becomes blocked, the muscle it supplies dies.

Left main artery

Circumflex artery

Right artery

Left anterior descending artery

the blood out and into the aorta, the body's major artery, and then by expanding to draw blood in from the veins. This pumping action occurs because the heart muscle is stimulated by electrical impulses that occur 60 to 100 times a minute. These electrical impulses are controlled from centers in the heart itself and also by the central nervous system. When your doctor takes an electrocardiogram (EKG), he or she is measuring these electrical impulses.

Stress and heart disease

Stress seems to cause heart disease in several ways. The adrenal hormones cortisol and epinephrine are released when your body undergoes stress. These hormones have both direct and indirect effects on your heart. Cortisol raises your blood pressure by causing your kidneys to retain more salt and fluid. This increases the amount of blood circulating through your cardiovascular system and so increases your blood pressure. At the same time that it causes you to retain salt, cortisol causes your kidneys to excrete more potassium in the urine. Not only does this imbalance exaggerate the action of salt on blood pressure, but it also can cause erratic heart rhythm. How? The interaction between salt and potassium in the heart muscle is part of what generates the electrical impulses that keep the heart beating.

Excess epinephrine, such as the amounts produced when you chronically overreact to stressful stimuli, can actually injure heart muscle by causing it to contract too hard to the point where the fibers can tear.

Both epinephrine and cortisol can increase the stickiness of platelets, a blood component that aids in coagulation or clotting. This increased clotting is life-saving when you're injured and might hemorrhage. If you're not losing blood, though, these sticky platelets can clump together and stick to the arterial walls. There the platelets can stimulate the growth of the muscle cells that line the arteries. Cholesterol circulating in the blood can attach to these cells and stimulate their growth. This sort of buildup of blood fats and fibrous tissue on the arterial walls is called plaque. As the plaque collects, the opening of the artery narrows, forcing the blood to push through a smaller opening. This buildup is called atherosclerosis and greatly increases the risk of heart disease, hypertension, stroke, and kidney disease. In fact, complications arising from atherosclerosis are the major cause of death in the United States. Atherosclerosis may occur with or without high blood pressure, although high blood pressure greatly increases your risk of developing it.

Stress and cholesterol

Stress hormones can also raise your blood cholesterol levels, adding to the problem. If you eat a high fat or high cholesterol diet or smoke (which also raises cholesterol), you may be setting the stage for serious cardiovascular illness. Atherosclerosis in the coronary arteries that supply the heart with blood may eventually narrow them to the point where the blood flow doesn't bring enough oxygen to the heart. This causes the chest pain known as angina. Angina is usually triggered by exertion and sometimes also by cold, but it may even occur during sleep. A more severe cut-off in blood supply to the heart muscle can so starve it of

High blood pressure and atherosclerosis

High blood pressure can injure a vessel's wall, causing breaks. Circulating platelets rush to the injury and stick to the vessel's wall. Fats in the circulating blood attach to the platelets, harden, and form plaque—which narrows the blood vessel. This build-up, called atherosclerosis, can lead to heart attack.

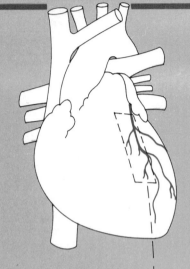

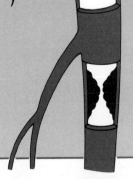

Vessel injured from high blood pressure

Fat deposits collect and form plaques of cholesterol

Fatty proteins and debris can harden

How Type A behavior was identified

Many of the most important discoveries in science and medicine seem to have been made almost by chance. So it was with Type A behavior.

One day, a workman made a chance remark that changed the way doctors look at heart disease. He was working in the waiting room of Drs. Friedman and Rosenman. "You know, there's something funny about the doctors' patients," he said. "Look at the front of these chairs. These weren't reupholstered so long ago. The backs look fine, but the seats are worn down to their threads! Something must keep these people on the edge of their seats," he laughed.

The workman's comment started wheels turning in the doctors' minds: what was it about their patients that made them unable to relax and sit back in their chairs? Was there some connection between this and their heart problems?

Yes, there was. Drs. Friedman and Rosenman had identified Type A behavior, now acknowledged by most specialists to be a major factor in heart disease.

oxygen that some part of the muscle dies. This is what is commonly called a heart attack, myocardial infarction, or coronary.

Hypertension with or without atherosclerosis can cause a disease called congestive heart failure. This occurs when the heart, which has enlarged like any other muscle asked to take on more work, can no longer pump effectively. Abnormal heart rates, where the heart rhythm may become fast or slow or wildly erratic, are another possible complication.

Type A behavior

Constant stress causes some people to bristle with aggressiveness and hostility, even though they may often hide its outward signs. You know the type. These people always seem impatient—waiting in traffic or supermarket lines seems like torture to them. They're constantly looking at their watches, tapping their feet, talking loudly, and doing many things at one time. You can't imagine them ever relaxing. Even when they're having fun, there's something angry about them. Whatever they're doing, they like to compete with someone. They're ambitious. They live to get ahead. In fact, modern life seems to encourage these people. People who talk and act fast, work obsessively, and do several things at once tend to get promoted over those who live life at a more human pace.

You probably won't be surprised to learn that people who behave in this harried way are more prone to health problems. In fact, they have double the risk of heart disease, the nation's number one killer. Their behavior has a name—type A, or coronary-prone, behavior. It was identified and named in the late 1950s by Drs. Meyer Friedman and Ray Rosenman, two cardiologists.

Friedman and Rosenman felt that the increase in heart disease since the beginning of the century was partly related to the stress of living in and having to adapt to an increasingly complex world. This type of environment, they say, has encouraged the development of Type A behavior.

Type A's are "aggressively involved in an incessant struggle to achieve more and more in less time," say Friedman and Rosenman. On top of having to do things faster, Type A's also have to struggle with obsta-

Mitral valve prolapse

Approximately one in ten women but fewer men have an unusual heart abnormality that often causes no symptoms but can be aggravated by stress. This condition is called mitral valve prolapse (MVP) and is caused by a malfunctioning valve between the upper and lower left chambers of the heart. Normally this valve should shut tightly when the heart contracts to pump blood, but in some people this valve balloons up (prolapses) into the lower chamber, causing blood to leak from the upper chamber.

When symptoms do occur, the person usually feels fluttering or pain in the chest that isn't related to exertion, fatigue, or shortness of breath. These symptoms tend to flare up in the presence of stress hormones.

Smoking and caffeine consumption can add to the problem.

Interestingly, MVP also often appears in women who are afflicted with panic disorders such as claustrophobia (an extreme fear of being closed in) and agoraphobia (an extreme fear of open, usually public, places), although this connection is not yet understood.

If you're bothered by these symptoms, have them checked out. Your doctor can usually diagnose MVP with a stethoscope, although sometimes he or she will use a painless ultrasound test called an echocardiogram. Most cases of MVP pose no danger, and you won't have to alter your activities at all. More severe cases may require medication such as beta blockers.

Because the mitral valve doesn't close tightly, blood leaks back into the left atrium instead of being pushed out into the body.

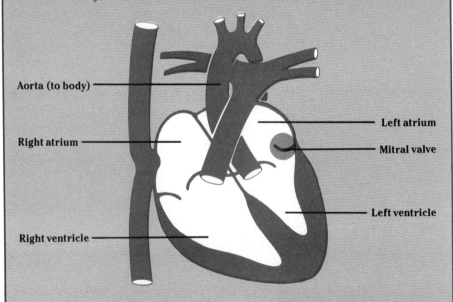

Aorta (to body)

Right atrium

Right ventricle

Left atrium

Mitral valve

Left ventricle

cles presented by people who don't necessarily see things their way.

A sense of control is of paramount importance to Type A's. No one puts in more effort on tasks they think they can cope with. On the other hand, Type A's are often more willing to throw in the towel on projects they feel they can't control, because the feeling of not being in control is so stressful to them.

Type A behavior can increase epinephrine release and also the amount of fats in the blood. These two factors, as we have seen, can play important roles in the development of heart disease.

Type A has an opposite—Type B. These people make better friends because they have more time for friendship. They value companionship and hobbies and relaxation for their own merits. Type Bs aren't unambitious or lazy, but they do place a lot less value on the outward signs of success. Type Bs don't have to feel that they're right all the time. They're guided much more by an inner sense of their own worth. Type Bs are less self-involved but more self-confident.

Are you a Type A?
Answer *agree* or *disagree* to the following questions to see whether you act like a Type A.

1. I'm bothered when people don't see things my way.

2. There's never enough time in a day.

3. When I'm mad I swear.

4. I often interrupt when people are talking because some people never seem to get to the point.

5. I like to do things quickly. I hate to waste time.

6. It's hard for me to just sit around and do nothing.

7. Sometimes I feel guilty because I have so little time to spend with my family and friends, but I can't change that for the moment.

If you had three or more *agree* answers, chances are you fall into the Type A behavior category.

If you took the Type A quiz and found that you show signs of Type A behavior, relax! Recent studies have shown that even severe Type A's can learn to modify their behavior and learn new responses to stress that are less dangerous to their health. These include learning to use the relaxation response, meditation, or biofeedback training. Read on to learn more about these.

Cancer

Researchers at the Albert Einstein College of Medicine in New York have found that stress can encourage tumor growth. Using mice that have been injected with cancerous cells capable of growing into a deadly tumor, they then subjected the animals to various stressors. Tumor cells seemed to thrive and grow more quickly in these stressed animals, because some of the chemicals released during the stress response seem to nourish the cancerous cells.

The presence of cancerous cells in your body causes a stress response. Your body attempts to cope with the cancer by producing a defensive inflammatory response around the cancerous cells. This defensive response is supposed to isolate the cancer so that it doesn't spread into the rest of the body. However, this defense reaction doesn't seem to work correctly against cancerous cells, because the inflammation brings more blood to the tumor, allowing it to grow and thrive. As you remember, stress causes the release of epinephrine, or adrenaline, a hormone that causes a rise in blood sugar. This means that the increased blood supply coming to the tumor is rich with sugars—just the food that the tumor needs to keep on growing. Other adrenal stress hormones also help nourish the growing tumor.

To make matters worse, the chemicals produced during stress act directly to suppress the action of the thymus gland and the lymphatic system, both of which are involved in fighting off invaders. So cancerous cells set off a vicious cycle in your body. Their very presence causes stress, and the release of the usual stress hormones encourages their growth, which causes more stress hormones to be released. The emotional stress of having cancer as well as the stress of treatment also contributes to this vicious cycle.

Using their theory that stress actually aids in tumor growth, the researchers at Einstein investigated whether they could slow a tumor's growth by suppressing the body's stress response. They hoped that by preventing the stress-induced enlargement of the adrenal gland and its increased activity or by preventing the shrinkage of the thymus and its decreased immune activity, they might be able to rob the tumor cells of their advantage.

Although these researchers' work is in a highly experimental stage on animals, their findings have generated some excitement in the cancer world. They found several substances that seemed to diminish these physical changes and helped the body fight back. One of these is beta-carotene, Vitamin A as it's found in vegetables and fruits. While they don't advocate beta-carotene as a cancer cure, they suggest that it might help conventional cancer therapies to work better.

Asthma

Asthma means "panting" in Greek. People who have asthma have attacks of severe breathing difficulty due to the narrowing of their airways. Asthma attacks may be brought on by allergies, irritants in the air, colds, exposure to cold air—or by stress. Stress doesn't cause asthma by itself, but it can trigger an attack in people who already have the disease. Some specialists say that people who suffer from asthma tend to have attacks when they're asked to cope with too much.

Sometimes, learning relaxation techniques and breath control can help asthmatics breathe more easily and can reduce the frequency of their attacks. However, people with this disorder must have asthma medication with them at all times. Stress management alone cannot prevent asthma attacks.

Hyperventilation

"Sometimes when I'm feeling very anxious, I get this awful feeling that I can't get my breath and that I may be going to die. If it's a bad day, I also get chest pains and feel dizzy."

This person is probably reacting to things that upset or frighten her by hyperventilating, or overbreathing. Many people do this without even knowing it. They feel like they're starving for air while they're actually taking in too much.

Learning why you have the frightening symptoms that come with hyperventilating can go a long way toward relieving them.

Practicing deep breathing exercises regularly may help you when you're under pressure.

Deep breathing

Learn to breathe rhythmically while staring at a fixed object. Try to establish a rhythm to your breathing by counting: for example, "in 2, 3, 4; out, 2, 3, 4." Keep the pace slow. When you've established a comfortable, relaxing rhythm, concentrate on feeling a little more relaxed with each exhalation. Focus on how you feel as you relax—weightless, pulsating, tingling, warm, or heavy.

Controlling hyperventilation

If you see someone hyperventilating, get a paper bag (not a plastic bag) and have the person hold the bag over the nose and mouth and breathe into the bag until breathing becomes normal. Breathing into a bag returns a high percentage of carbon dioxide to the lungs, helping to produce a normal breathing cycle.

Where's your weakness?

While almost everyone feels some amount of stress, not everyone has the same physical reactions. For example, some people will get headaches, others heartburn. In some people, stress and ulcers go together. Whether or not stress causes ulcers, it obviously doesn't help anyone who develops an ulcer.

Ulcers

"This job is giving me ulcers!" is a common refrain but sometimes it has a ring of truth. Stress often plays a role in the development of ulcers. In fact, ulcers are one of the stress diseases originally identified by Dr. Hans Selye, the father of the stress syndrome. Ulcers are small sores that form in the lining of the stomach and small intestine. You may have heard of gastric ulcers (in the stomach itself) and duodenal ulcers (in the duodenum, the beginning of the small intestine where the stomach empties).

Since no one knows exactly how or why ulcers form, no one knows exactly how stress can pave the way for them. Sometimes stress and anxiety cause an ulcer by making the stomach manufacture more acid, and this acid may eat away at the stomach's lining. However,

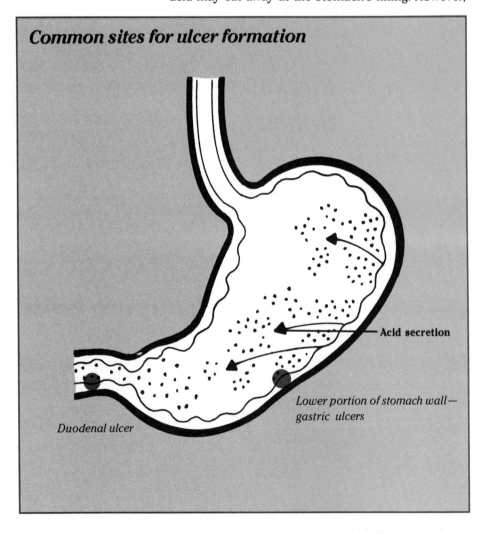

Common sites for ulcer formation

Acid secretion

Lower portion of stomach wall—
gastric ulcers

Duodenal ulcer

many ulcer patients don't have increased acid secretions; many have decreased acid secretions.

Even though the connection isn't fully understood, doctors often advise their ulcer patients to avoid stress as much as possible. People with ulcers are generally given a drug like Tagamet that actually slows down acid secretion. Your doctor may also advise you to eat smaller meals.

Headaches

Eric Baldwin, a 33-year-old computer programmer and father of three, developed a troubling headache. Intermittent at first, it began to show up daily. After suffering these headaches for several months, he went to his doctor, afraid that he might have a serious disease like hypertension or a brain tumor.

His doctor decided to do some testing and sent him for an EEG (which measures the electrical activity of different parts of the brain), X rays of his sinuses, and blood tests. As she expected, the tests showed nothing abnormal. "Eric, I'm not making light of your headaches," she said, "but I can't find anything obviously wrong. Usually in cases like this, the headaches are caused by stress. Are you under any particular pressures?" And out came Eric's tale of woe: he felt that he had come to a dead end in his job. The office was using his considerable computer talents but not promoting him. Around the time the headaches began, Eric had been so angry he had thought about moving to another company. His marriage wasn't going too smoothly, either. He and his wife weren't fighting, but the pressures of bringing up 6-year-old twins and a new baby and having two careers left them with little time for communication of any sort. Eric felt burned-out; his life seemed hopeless, and the dull pain of his headaches seemed to reinforce his feelings of despair.

"I'd say you have a lot going on," said his doctor sympathetically. "From what you've said, I think that stress is at the root of your problem." And she told him how stress can cause headaches.

Headaches are complicated disorders with numerous causes, but to simplify matters, we can reduce headaches to two basic types. One is caused by contractions (dilations) of blood vessels in the scalp. This type of headache is called a vascular, or migraine,

Headache ahead

Some psychologists say that people who need to feel in control suffer from headaches because they can't control everything. The realization that they don't really have control a lot of the time keeps this type of person in a perpetual alarm state. The hormones needed to maintain the alarm reaction can cause the blood vessels of the head to constrict and the muscles of the head, neck, and shoulders to tighten, bringing on a headache.

Caffeine headaches

If you're a coffee, tea, or soda drinker who has tried to stop drinking these beverages altogether, you've undoubtedly suffered from a caffeine headache. Mildly addictive, caffeine enlarges the blood vessels in your head. If you stop your caffeine intake or reduce it radically, your vessels contract, causing a headache. Caffeine headaches can be incapacitating, and they don't respond well to aspirin. What your system needs—you've guessed it— is caffeine. If you want to reduce your caffeine intake, try cutting back slowly.

headache. The other type of headache is caused by sustained muscle tension in the forehead, neck, or scalp. This type of headache is called a tension headache.

Headaches are one of the commonest symptoms of an overload of psychological stress. People often say, "That gives me a headache" or "What a pain in the neck" when referring to situations or people that tax their abilities to cope.

Certain personality types are more prone to headaches than others. As you would expect, Type A's have more headaches, and the more strongly A a person is, the more likely he or she is to have both types of headache.

The chemicals in cigarettes and alcohol can give you a headache, so smoking and drinking are particularly bad ways of coping with stress if you're headache-prone.

Treatment for muscle tension headaches involves aspirin, occasionally muscle relaxants, heat, and gentle massage of the scalp, neck, and shoulders. If you suffer often from vascular headaches, your doctor may want to treat you with specific antimigraine drugs. Relaxation techniques and biofeedback are particularly effective long-term treatments for headaches.

Dental problems

Stress can send you to your dentist. We often carry our tension in our jaws. Look at some of the tense or Type A people whom you know, and you'll probably notice that several of them are unconsciously clenching their jaws when they're tense—and even when they think they're relaxing. How does your own jaw feel?

Florence Chen, a waitress in a Chicago luncheonette, was bothered off and on by tired facial muscles, particularly those around the left side of her jaw. She also suffered from headaches and occasional ear pain that troubled her enough to visit her doctor. He could find nothing wrong and suggested her symptoms were probably due to tension. The headaches and facial pain continued, and several months later Florence also began to hear strange popping noises and to have trouble opening her mouth wide. The facial pains began to get worse.

When Florence saw her dentist for a routine checkup, she complained about her symptoms. Her dentist told her about a jaw disorder called temporo-mandibular joint pain-syndrome, or TMJ. (It's also known as myofacial pain-dysfunction syndrome.) The symptoms the dentist described were very much like those she had been suffering. He said that this syndrome can come from a faulty bite or injury but that most commonly it comes from stress.

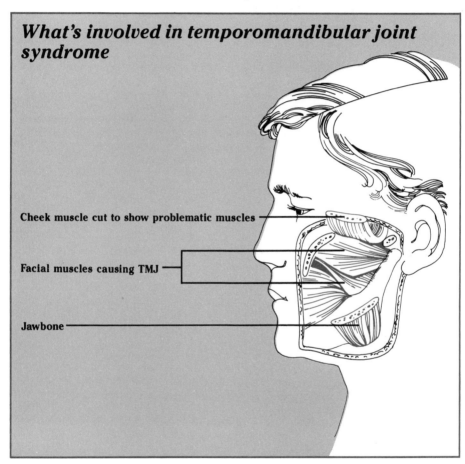

What's involved in temporomandibular joint syndrome

Cheek muscle cut to show problematic muscles

Facial muscles causing TMJ

Jawbone

The best treatment for TMJ is warm compresses on the jaw, aspirin, and exercises to relax the jaw. If these simple measures don't work, your dentist can fit you for a device to wear when you sleep that will relax the muscle spasms around your jaw. Some dentists may also prescribe mild tranquilizers to help you relax. Others feel that tranquilizers don't really help you cope with the stress that is causing your tension and discourage their use.

Bruxism

Stress may also cause you to grind your teeth so much that you actually wear them down. This common condition is called bruxism. Many people do their tooth grinding at night and aren't even aware of the problem until their dentist examines their teeth and notices its effects.

Relaxation techniques are commonly prescribed to help patients with bruxism. Your dentist can also fit you with a type of splint that will protect your teeth from damage.

Depression and anxiety

Depression and anxiety are common by-products of too much stress. In fact, many more people may develop emotional symptoms from too much stress than develop physical problems. Typical psychological effects of too much stress include:

- Fatigue

- Lowered sex drive

- Difficulty in concentrating

- Difficulty in making decisions.

Fatigue that you can't get rid of with one or two good nights' sleep is one of the most common signs of too much stress. Fatigue is also a common symptom of depression. Overcoming this sort of fatigue involves identifying the stressors in your life and learning new ways of coping with them. One of the best ways to overcome fatigue is exercising regularly. This will also help relieve some of the other symptoms of stress overload such as depression and nervousness.

- Exercise gets your circulation going and increases blood flow to your brain. It also strengthens your muscles so that day-to-day life is less of an effort. Many doctors are now prescribing exercise to treat depression and anxiety.

- Lowered sex drive is also a very common sign of both too much stress and depression. It's a by-product of an overall low energy level. Satisfying sexual relations are an important stress reducer. Strained sexual relations are stressful and add to your overall stress level. Fortunately, sex drive usually returns promptly once you've found techniques for managing the stress in your life.

• Difficulty in concentrating and in making decisions is a subtle side effect that many people don't even associate with being under stress. They just think they don't have enough will power and try to push on anyway. Sometimes when your mind seems to slow down, speed up, or go in several directions at once, it's just indicating that you're trying to deal with too much all at once. Try taking a mini-vacation. Give yourself a day in which you don't have to do anything. Try to keep your mind off your worries. Try to get some physical activity, because this will revitalize you, but don't push yourself. This is your time to unwind. You'll be surprised to find how your perspective can change from just a day or a weekend off. Don't be surprised to find that what looked like an impossible decision to make or an impossible pile of work to finish has shrunken to a much more manageable size, because you're confronting it from a more relaxed, distanced perspective.

Infectious diseases

Have you ever wondered why you often get colds or fever blisters or other contagious disorders just when you're trying hard to cope with some new pressure—a new job, income taxes, getting married? Most of us have probably had this happen. It's the proverbial "last straw" arriving at precisely the wrong time.

This bad timing results from the effects of stress hormones on the immune system. One way these stress hormones may make you sick is by decreasing the numbers or depressing the functioning of the invasion-fighting cells that circulate in your blood. Normally, these immune system cells continually sweep your body on the lookout for invaders. Most of the time they make quick work of these foreign cells, and you never even know they were in your body.

Sometimes, however, invaders overpower your defenses, either because so many of them appear all at once or because your defenses aren't working up to par because of the effect of stress hormones. These hormones seem to weaken your immune system directly.

When you're sick
Sometimes, no matter what you do, the flu temporarily defeats your immune system's defenses, and you come down with a sore throat and runny nose. Slow down! You can't expect your body to cope with a major stressor and fight the bug simultaneously. You'll get well faster if you give your body a break, and rest. This doesn't necessarily mean that you have to stay in bed. See how much you feel like doing, and let that be your guide. Whatever you do, don't be an extreme Type A and press on, ignoring your body's pleas for rest.

The bad and the good

Stress worsens your ability to cope with some diseases, as you've seen. Hypertension, certain heart diseases, cancer, backache, headache, some breathing problems, ulcers—all are complicated by stress. When you add serious fatigue, lowered sex drive, and reduced concentration abilities to the list, you've got a lot of problems linked to stress. What's the good news? You can manage stress, which the upcoming pages will help you do.

Stress and sickness

Stress can increase your susceptibility to illness by disrupting your immune system. What can you do to protect yourself? In addition to the techniques you've read about, you can turn to meditation, exercise, and biofeedback—whichever you find attractive. Counterbalance the stress with these stress reducers.

Stress and loneliness

Stress and loneliness can also weaken your resistance to infection. A group of researchers at Ohio State University found that the students they tested had the highest resistance to cold sores right after summer vacation, when they were well rested. Students who tested out to be lonely and less involved with friends had lower resistance to cold sores.

As Holmes and Rahe predicted, mourning and the emotions that accompany it can change your resistance to disease. Many people know someone who became very ill soon after the death of someone close. A recent report from the Mount Sinai School of Medicine in New York showed that the immune system of recently widowed men was weakened for several months after the wife's death. Another study showed that depressed people had weakened immune systems. The researchers again concluded that this decreased immune system function was caused by high levels of cortisol and other hormones that suppress the body's defenses.

At stressful times, you should be particularly careful to use some of the stress management techniques described on page xx. Meditation, exercise, biofeedback training, and other ways to tone down your body's response to stress can help you avoid illness at these times.

Back pain

Back pain has plagued people ever since we began to walk upright. Few people will escape back pain at some point in their life. Of course, back pain may be traceable to an actual injury to the spine or its muscles and ligaments, but as any orthopedist will tell you, many cases of back pain have no obvious cause. Many experts feel that psychological stress underlies a large number of the cases of unexplained back pain that they see each day.

The stress response, when kept up over a long time, finally causes the muscles of the back to clamp up into a chronic spasm that causes you pain. This sort of pain seems to occur mainly in the neck, shoulders, and lower back, the parts of your spine that move the most. You can also get a backache if your muscles clamp up as a result of a sudden alarm reaction.

Preventing stress-related back pain

If you have chronic back pain that doctors can't find a physical cause for, your pain is probably stress-related. The best way to treat this condition is also the best way to prevent it. You need to lessen the tension you're holding in your back and learn ways of coping with emotional stress other than transferring it into your body. Acupuncture, massage, meditation, biofeedback, and swimming are useful. If your back isn't currently hurting, you may want to start a special back exercise program to relax and strengthen your muscles. Of course, if you have back pain from time to time, check with your doctor before starting any exercise program. Not all back problems are alike, and what might be great for one type of back problem might pose problems for another.

If you have back pain, aspirin often will help relieve the pain enough for you to move about. Warm showers directed at your back or a long, relaxing soak in the tub can help, too. More severe cases of back pain may require up to two weeks of bed rest. Investing in a firm mattress or getting a bed board (½ inch plywood will do fine) can help you considerably. The firmer support allows your back muscles to relax while you sleep, rather than staying tense as they try to maintain your position on a saggy mattress.

Back pain and stress

Back problems and weak support muscles often go together. Strain on weak muscles can make them spasm, or contract, causing pain. Usually, tensed muscles are slow to relax, and the pain lingers on. Exercise can help in two ways: it strengthens the support muscles, reducing the strain on them, and it relieves your stress and tension, making relaxation easier for you.

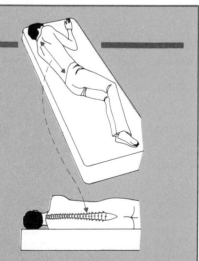

Posture for your back
Keep your back properly aligned while you sleep. Keeping your knees partially bent helps align your back.

Back relaxers

Do these exercises gently and slowly. Stop if they cause pain.

1. Lie on your back, arms straight out on the floor from your shoulders, knees to your chest, and roll your hips gently from side to side.

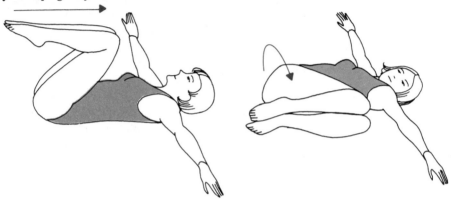

2. Lie on your back, legs straight out. Bend one knee to your chest and grasp the knee and heel of that leg. Move your leg gently, so that you can feel your hip rotating in its socket. Repeat on the other side.

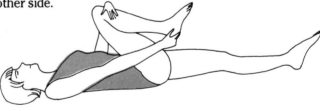

3. Lie on your back with your knees drawn up as in #1. Hold this position and breathe deeply.

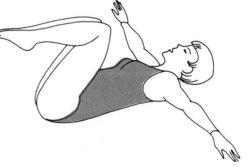

4. Bent-knee sit-ups help your back by strengthening your stomach muscles so that your back doesn't get pulled out of alignment by a sagging middle. To do these, lie with your torso flat on the floor, your knees bent, your arms against your sides, palms flat on the floor. Lift your trunk to a sitting position, almost touching your chest to your knees. You'll make maximum use of your stomach muscles if you gently roll your head and then shoulders as you lift off the ground. Then roll slowly back down. Start with two repetitions and work up to 25 by adding only two more each day.

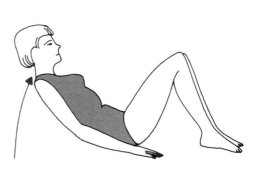

5. Sit in a chair, feet about a foot apart. Slowly roll forward from your waist so that your face rests between your knees and your arms hang toward the floor, then slowly roll back up, feeling each vertebra as it rolls back up against the chair. Sit tall, stretch up, and then roll forward again and repeat. This is an exercise that you can do several times a day, even in an office.

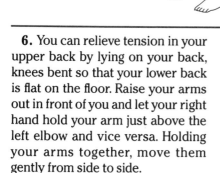
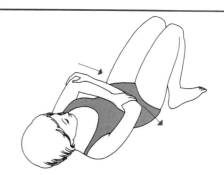

6. You can relieve tension in your upper back by lying on your back, knees bent so that your lower back is flat on the floor. Raise your arms out in front of you and let your right hand hold your arm just above the left elbow and vice versa. Holding your arms together, move them gently from side to side.

Dangerous stress

Unfortunately, many doctors and most accident victims regard accidents as just that—accidents. Because of this tendency, victims of accidents may have difficulty getting the help they need. Yet accidents are the leading cause of death in the young and a major cause of death at any age.

Accidentitis

When you're under stress, watch out for accidents. This may seem like odd advice, but an increasing amount of research has shown a clear relationship between stress and accidents. Some people possibly have accidents the way others develop diseases. Like getting sick, having an accident may serve to take some of the pressure off for a while and allow you to relax and get the rest you need.

You've probably heard someone say that another person is "accident prone." It used to be thought that there was an "accident-prone" personality, which was impulsive, full of buried anger, and needful of immediate gratification. Newer research has displaced some of these ideas. "Accidentitis" may be a response to a stress overload.

In a study of drivers involved in fatal car accidents, one researcher found that 20 percent of these people had had an upsetting or stressful incident within six hours of the accident. Another study showed that many car accident victims were faced with some sort of threatening life transition. In many cases, the accidents were preceded by extreme tension and hostile behavior such as brawling, drinking, and truancy.

Unfortunately, many doctors and most accident victims regard accidents as just that—accidents. Because of this tendency, victims of accidents may have difficulty getting the help they need. Yet accidents are the leading cause of death in the young and a major cause of death at any age.

Doctors who study accident proneness know that people who have repeated accidents need therapy to help them find better outlets for their tension and to learn effective ways of coping with stress.

5 Stress management

You don't have to fall victim to stress diseases. Even though you may be living through major life changes, such as a death in the family or problems in your children's lives, you can cope. Even though you may live in a stressful environment like a crowded, polluted city, you can cope. You can cope without changing your life circumstances; indeed, basic changes may not always be possible.

You can change how your body reacts to stressors. Of course, you won't be able to rid yourself completely of stress reactions, but you can, with practice, learn to react less to the smaller stresses of daily life. Occasionally things will still come out of the blue and throw you for a loop, but you can learn to help your body react less strongly even to these stressors. Many doctors now believe that modifying your body's response to stress can help prevent or slow down the development of many stress-related diseases.

Your two basic stress choices

While you can't remove all environmental, personal, and work stressors, you have the choice of receiving them directly or using stress management techniques to protect yourself. The probable consequences of your choice are shown below.

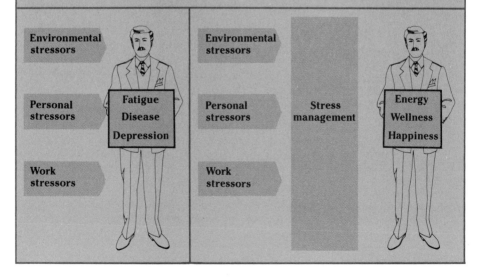

Environmental stressors		Environmental stressors	
Personal stressors	Fatigue Disease Depression	Personal stressors	Stress management	Energy Wellness Happiness
Work stressors		Work stressors		

Handling stress

One of the most important things to realize is that you have choices in handling stress. Although your physical response to stress is automatic, you can teach yourself how to let things roll off your back. This way, the state of your emotions is less likely to affect your body's health. More and more, doctors realize that the best treatment for stress isn't tranquilizers, which only treat some of the symptoms, but reducing your reactions to stress.

Oxygen! Oxygen!

The last thing you may want to hear when you're under pressure is "Take a deep breath!" But this well-meant advice works better than you might think. Many of us, when stressed, don't breathe properly. We take the short, shallow breaths of the fight or flight response—some of us even hold our breath. Since all the tissues of our body need oxygen in order to function, poor breathing can leave us feeling fatigued, dizzy, and upset.

Some of the stress reduction techniques given here will appeal to you while others may not. Some, such as deep breathing and passive relaxation, are appropriate for use at the very moment of stress; others, such as exercise and meditation, are to be used daily to reduce the muscular tension and stress hormone output that can lead you to overreact to daily stressors. Choose ones that seem natural and comfortable to you so that you'll use them daily and incorporate them into your routine. If meditating doesn't appeal to you, maybe you'd prefer having a daily swim or learning to use biofeedback.

You may need to ease yourself into certain stress management techniques. For instance, you may find exercise difficult at first but—providing you have your doctor's go-ahead—an exercise program that you start slowly will eventually pay off, and you'll feel increasingly better. Occasionally, you'll have to miss your daily exercise. In that case, the relaxation response or self-hypnosis might be exactly what you need to stay calm.

Master the art of breathing

Taking a few deep breaths is one of the handiest tools we have for controlling anxiety right on the spot. No matter what's going on, if you can mentally stand back a moment and take a few breaths, you'll find that you feel calmer and more in control. "But I can't possibly stop and take a deep breath in the middle of some stressful situation like my boss yelling at me," you protest. Why not? Try taking that deep breath. You don't need any special equipment. Your boss won't notice anything, and you'll probably react more calmly to your boss's tirade. You may have heard the advice to count to ten before replying to someone who has made you angry. Apply that advice, and use those ten seconds to take a couple of deep, calming breaths before you react.

Singing can be an excellent stress reducer, because it takes advantage of the same kind of breath control. (It's also a good exercise.) If you enjoy singing, singing will be stress-reducing. Singing also forces you to take deep breaths, which help rid you of tension. Naturally, you can't let loose an aria when you're being chewed out at work, but you can sing in some situations where you may be boiling away with anger. Consider a few songs in the shower or as you walk or drive to work.

How to breathe

You're probably pretty sure you know how to breathe. You do it thousands of times every day. But there are certain deep breathing techniques that have been developed over the centuries by many different cultures, and these can go a long way toward helping you relax. Follow these instructions and practice the technique a few times a day. Eventually you'll learn to respond to emotional stress by breathing in this way rather than by going into an alarm reaction.

1. Deep breathing is a three-point rhythm. Start by sitting up straight and inhaling deeply from the bottom of your stomach below where your diaphragm begins. Let your stomach swell out as you slowly pull in air. Inhale slowly and think about the air getting from the bottom of your lungs near your waist to their very tops right under your shoulders. Let your chest swell.

2. If you feel a particular area of tension in your body, think about directing the flow of air to that part.

3. Hold in the nourishing air a moment or two and then let it out as slowly as you took it in. Your chest will lower, and your stomach will pull in. Use your stomach muscles to push out every last bit of air. Repeat until you're breathing comfortably in this calm, three-point rhythm.

4. As you become more comfortable with this technique, you'll find that you can breathe this way without thinking about all the steps. When you are in a pressured situation, rely on the calming effects of deep breaths even if your heart is pounding and you feel like yelling at whoever or whatever is upsetting you. Reacting from a state of inner calm will do far more for you in the long run than flying off the handle.

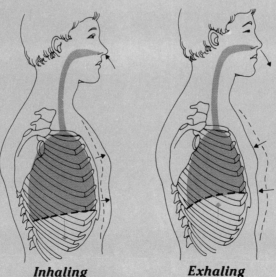

Inhaling   **Exhaling**

Learning to relax

Learning to relax takes practice. First, choose a slogan that you'll feel comfortable saying each time you practice—for example, "Ease up" or "Slow down." Or, if you prefer, use a short prayer. Then follow the steps shown here.

If you prefer, try this method: breathe out slowly while concentrating on a particular muscle. Imagine a wave of relaxation starting at the muscle and spreading out to the rest of your body.

No matter what method you choose, do it twice. Then return to whatever you were doing.

Do your relaxation exercise at least 10 times daily.

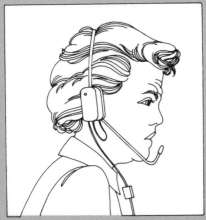

Stop whatever you're doing.

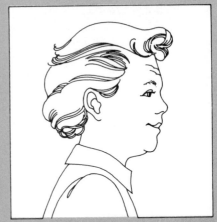

Smile—openly, if appropriate; otherwise, smile inwardly.

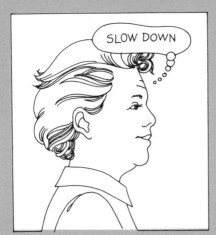

SLOW DOWN

Say your relaxation slogan to yourself.

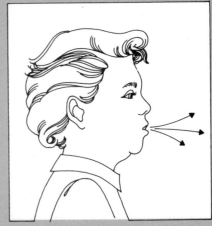

Breathe out slowly. As you do, think about how relaxed you're feeling.

Mectitation

The quest for relief from stress has led many to take up various forms of relaxation techniques long practiced in the East. The most popular of these is transcendental meditation (TM). Many scientists claim that the meditative process relieves nervous system stress even more efficiently than dreaming or sleeping.

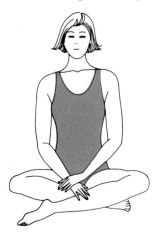

Calm away your stress

Here's an antidote to all the stress hormones that you churn up during a day of seemingly constant fight or flight responses. Where fight or flight is automatic and hyper, its antidote is a relaxation technique that must be learned and practiced. While you may not always be able to apply this antidote right on the spot, practicing ways of relaxing for a set period every day will eventually help you react less strongly to the minor stresses of daily life. This antidote has many different names and uses many different induction techniques, but all counter the effects of stress:

- Transcendental meditation

- The relaxation response

- Progressive relaxation.

Meditation

Meditation was introduced on a large scale to this country during the 1960s. The form of meditation most Americans have been exposed to is transcendental meditation, or TM. TM is an adaptation of many ancient meditative techniques of the East. It was invented by an Indian guru, the Maharishi Mahesh Yogi, who felt that most Westerners were put off by the long religious training and extraordinary body control needed to master many of the traditional meditation techniques and were therefore denied the benefits of meditation. The Maharishi dispensed with most of the spiritual trappings and came up with a simple technique that can be practiced once or twice a day for twenty minutes. The meditator sits quietly in a comfortable position and repeats a word known as a mantra. This word is picked especially for you by your TM teacher, and you repeat it over and over to help tune out distracting thoughts.

TM caught on quickly. People said that it made them feel calmer and happier and gave them more energy. Soon enough, open-minded doctors realized that TM might be good for more than the soul. Dr. Herbert Benson, a cardiologist at Harvard Medical School, was the first to make thorough studies of meditators. He found that TM has many very beneficial physical effects. It lowers heart rate and oxygen consumption, two things that happen normally when you're asleep. TM also increases alpha brain wave activity. (Your brain puts out alpha waves when you're relaxed and alert but not asleep.) Meditators had generally low blood pressure and low levels of lactate, a by-product of muscle use that can build up in our blood and make us feel anxious. Meditation seems to counteract the physiological changes of the fight or flight response by putting the body into an alert, relaxed state. Dr. Benson realized that these changes weren't unique to meditation. They were part of a general response that our bodies can learn to make to counteract stress. He called this the Relaxation Response.

The relaxation response

Dr. Benson went even further than the Maharishi in simplifying the techniques of the relaxation response. His technique has four components:

• A quiet environment: try to meditate in a quiet room or in a spot outdoors where you know you won't be disturbed. Some people go to a church to help them shut out the noises of the external world. As you become more practiced, you'll be able to meditate wherever you are.

Select a mantra

A mantra is a sound that you repeat—no meaning necessary. By repeating your mantra, you keep thoughts and distractions from interrupting or stressing you. Repeating the mantra also calms many people, relaxing the mind and body. Once you select a mantra and use it a few times, you'll find that turning to it automatically calms you.

• A mental device: in traditional meditative forms you chant sounds like *om*—a mantra—to help you focus your concentration and tune out distracting thoughts. The same is true when you're eliciting the relaxation response, but you can use any short word that comes to mind. Many people use words like *one* or *peace*. You can say the word aloud or to yourself each time you breathe out.

• A passive attitude: your meditation time is when you should let your mind relax and stop the ceaseless struggle to think or figure things out. Inevitably, distracting thoughts will come into your mind when you're starting to meditate. Instead of worrying about them, just let them float away. Don't pay any attention to them, and don't worry that you're having them. Use your meditation word to help you push these distractions from your mind.

Since you may worry about time passing while you're meditating, set a kitchen timer and put it far enough away that you don't hear its ticking. This way, you won't have to keep stopping and glancing at your watch. You'll know to stay with the relaxation response until the timer rings.

• A comfortable position: you don't have to crank yourself into the traditional (and for many Westerners uncomfortable) Lotus position. If you're not comfortable enough, you won't be able to stop thinking about your discomfort and your muscles will tense up. However, if you're too comfortable, you might fall asleep, so don't try to meditate lying down. Sit comfortably. Or if you find walking relaxing, you might even want to walk in slow circles for the duration of your meditation.

Progressive relaxation

Here's another useful stress management technique that you can use to calm yourself and blunt your reaction to a stressful situation. The beauty of progressive relaxation is that you can use it wherever you are without anyone's noticing.

Sit or lie down in a quiet place. Starting at your toes, tense a body part and then consciously release the tension from that part, telling it to be soft and free of tension. Work your way slowly up your body, right to your scalp. Again, be sure to keep a passive attitude. This is not the time to worry about what you have to buy at the store. If thoughts intrude, and you find that you're tensing again, go back and rerelax any tight muscles. When you feel you're relaxed all over, try to stay in this calm state. Give yourself this ten- or fifteen-minute break in which you're completely off the hook. You'll be surprised at how good you feel when you've finished.

Hypnosis

Self-hypnosis

Hypnosis is a state of intense concentration. You can learn to hypnotize yourself and use your concentrating powers to reduce stress. While meditation requires time for self-orientation—sitting down, repeating your mantra, and readying yourself to relax—self-hypnosis takes only a couple of minutes.

Rebecca never dreamed that she or anyone she knew would ever be hypnotized. "When my doctor suggested that I learn self-hypnosis to help control my anxiety so I could stop smoking, I was shocked. I had always associated hypnosis with magic acts where they hypnotize someone who gets up and acts like a chicken! But my doctor said he thought I should check it out. So I did, and I'm very glad I listened to him. I was able to stop smoking over a month or so, and I continue to use hypnosis every day to help me with whatever tasks I have to do. Self-hypnosis has really made all the difference in my life."

Hypnosis is a state of intensely focused concentration that humans and animals share. Anytime you're focusing fixedly on something particular, you have entered a kind of hypnotic trance. But hypnosis doesn't have to be a random state. Hypnosis (where a therapist hypnotizes you) and self-hypnosis (where you hypnotize yourself) are actually extremely valuable and effective tools for habit control, relaxation, and time management. When you're hypnotized, you're more open to suggestions. If, when hypnotized, you tell yourself that you're going to stop smoking cigarettes or that you're calm and relaxed or that you're going to get down to work, you'll probably follow your instructions.

A hypnotherapist, psychiatrist, and many other types of health professionals can hypnotize you and then teach you how to hypnotize yourself. The technique is not difficult to learn. Successfully getting into the hypnotic state involves relaxing your mind and body and then receiving suggestions that you will go into a deeply focused, receptive state. Induction tech-

Three uses of hypnosis

You can use hypnosis to improve your concentration, which you can direct toward meeting challenges, changing habits, or solving problems. In each case, you'll need to plan your actions; then practice, order, or select; and follow through to success, change, or solution. Here's a summary of the three uses of hypnosis:

Meeting challenges	Habit changing	Problem solving
Plan	Plan	Plan
Rehearse	Set priorities	Select a solution
Succeed	Change	Solve

niques vary. Hypnosis is much like meditation except that you can hypnotize yourself within a couple of minutes or even less when you have some experience with the technique.

Three special uses

Hypnosis can be used to *rehearse*. If you're gearing up for a job interview, hypnotizing yourself and then actually rehearsing the interview and having it go well can be extremely helpful in reducing your anxiety and keeping you in control, thus increasing the probability of a successful interview.

Hypnosis can be used for *habit control*. Many therapists teach patients with addictions and bad habits to use self-hypnosis as the centerpiece of their treatment. When you're hypnotized, you or your therapist gives you a suggestion—for example, that you will not want to smoke anymore. Naturally, this won't work without your cooperation. You still may desire cigarettes very strongly and have to work hard to keep yourself away from them, but hypnosis has helped many people keep to their resolve.

Hypnosis is also used as a *relaxation tool*. You use it in much the same way that you use meditation to quiet your mind and focus deeply on your inner self. But unlike meditation, hypnosis is a state in which you're more likely to respond to suggestions.

Imaging techniques

It has been known to doctors since the 1920s that many cases of warts can be cured through hypnotic suggestion. Although this phenomenon has been the subject of numerous scientific studies over the years, no one knows exactly why it works. Most researchers believe that the hypnosis somehow permits you to generally boost your body's immune system enough to fight off the wart-causing virus.

From warts to cancer may seem like a major leap, but some doctors are using imaging techniques to boost the effects of traditional cancer therapies and to fight diseases such as rheumatoid arthritis and a variety of infections. This is not to suggest in any way that psychological techniques alone are sufficient to treat cancer, but imaging techniques can, in some instances, stimulate the immune system. Most doctors who use these psychological techniques along with a more conventional medication do so because they can't hurt and may help.

Some people can't relax because they don't understand how their bodies react to stress and what to do about it.

First, the patient is simply told about how the immune system functions. Then he or she is taught self-hypnosis or some other relaxation technique and is instructed to visualize the immune system working to fight off the invader. In the case of a cancer, the patient may try to imagine the immune system agents surrounding and fighting off the cancerous cells. He or she might visualize this as an actual battle.

Dr. Bernard Newton, a psychologist who heads the Newton Center for Clinical Hypnosis in Los Angeles, has studied the cases of 203 patients with advanced cancers who didn't respond to traditional treatments and were referred to his center. These patients were taught self-hypnosis and were instructed to develop strong images of their immune systems fighting off the cancer. They were also given hypnotic suggestions to help increase their feeling of being in control of their lives and to reduce negative feelings about their chances for survival. Of the 203 patients in the study, 54 percent of those who had been treated for at least 10 sessions in a three-month period were still alive at the time of the study, while only 11 percent of those who had fewer than 10 imaging sessions in the same time period were still alive. These differences in outcome were not linked to the severity of the disease, type of cancer, age, sex, or type of medical treatment. When Dr. Newton analyzed his results, he found that the people most likely to fight the cancer successfully were those who were able to respond positively and vividly without giving up.

Biofeedback

Some people find relaxing very difficult because they have no idea how tense and overwrought their bodies are. Biofeedback may help them get a sense of what their bodies are doing and how to slow down. Biofeedback is a fairly simple concept. It's a way of plugging into different systems of your body, listening to them, and using their feedback to monitor or learn to control them.

Biofeedback instruments are often used to help people learn when they're tense and how to relax. You're hooked up either to a machine that reads brain waves or muscular tension in one part of the body or to a machine that reads minute changes in the electricity of the skin that indicate tension. When the instrument reads that you're tense, a tone sounds. You're then instructed to make the tone go off by whatever

Biofeedback imaging exercise

Imagine your anxiety level being controlled by a volume knob that you can turn down to lower your body's reactivity to stress. You can do this exercise with or without a biofeedback machine. By pairing the image of turning down the volume knob with the actual physiological effort required to make the biofeedback tone drop, you can condition your body to relax as soon as you think about turning down the volume—even without hooking yourself up to the machine.

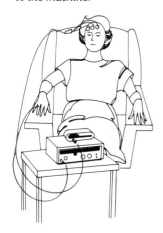

means you can. As you become more and more relaxed, the tone drops in volume until you turn it off completely. The tone makes the process of learning to relax much faster because it helps you monitor your progress. It teaches you just how your body feels when it isn't tensed up. A lot of people really can't identify this feeling. If true relaxation isn't just flopping down in front of a television set or having a drink, how does it feel? Biofeedback tools can help you tell. They can also help you learn just which situations or people or types of activity are stressful for you.

Physical responses

Migraine sufferers can be taught to control or partially control their pain by using biofeedback. Doctors who use this technique say it works because migraines are caused by contractions and dilations of blood vessels in the scalp. Lowering the blood flow through the veins relieves the pain because the blood doesn't press so hard against the blood vessel walls. The person is hooked up to a thermometer that records the temperature in his hands and prints it out for him to see. He is then told to concentrate on warming his hands. In quite a short time, with the use of feedback to tell him how well he's doing, he can learn to warm his hands by increasing the blood flowing through them—and thus he can relieve the pressure in the blood vessels of his scalp.

Biofeedback has also been used to help people control such physiological functions as blood pressure and stomach acid secretion.

Biofeedback used to be a laboratory technique. Today, you can buy numerous inexpensive biofeedback tools to use at home to help you learn how to control your tension. Look for them in catalogs of health and sports items.

Eliot Weiss, a traveling book salesman, recently found that a biofeedback machine helped him get his tension under control wherever he was. "Hooking myself up to this gadget isn't my idea of how to achieve oneness with the universe. I prefer to sit quietly and look at the mountains out my window or to run a couple of miles. But sometimes you don't have time to do things like that, or things leave you so frazzled that you can't seem to calm down no matter what. Then bi-

Relaxation tanks may offer you a way to stop smoking, cope with stress, and become more alert, clear-headed, and able to concentrate.

ofeedback tools like this are excellent, because they really do feed back your anxiety level to you and help you regulate it internally."

Relaxation tanks

If the idea of floating your cares away inside a tank of body-temperature water appeals to you, you might want to try one of the newer stress management tools: relaxation tanks. These tanks, which are like oversize bathtubs inside a small room, are designed to put you in a state of sensory deprivation, which means that all your senses are resting and not being used. You'll find absolute darkness inside a flotation tank, so your eyes don't have anything to do. The tank is well insulated, so your ears will hear nothing unless you splash or make some other noise. Once you get used to the smell of the epsom salts dissolved in the water to make you float, your nose has no more work. Since the water temperature is exactly that of your skin, you lose track of the boundary between your body and the water. The salts added to the water make you so buoyant that you don't have to make any effort to stay afloat. You just lie there fully relaxed.

Dr. Ovide Pomerleau, a stress management researcher at the University of Connecticut, says that for certain types of people, tanks may be a way to stop smoking, cope with stress, and generally become more alert, clear-headed, and able to concentrate. A hospital in Wisconsin did a study and found that relaxation tanks help people control headaches, chronic pain, anxiety, and ulcers, to name a few. Floating, like hard aerobic exercise and also like cigarette smoking and other stressors, stimulates endorphin release along with stress hormones. Endorphins are morphine-like substances that our bodies release with the stress hormones epinephrine, norepinephrine, and cortisol. Most cities now have relaxation tank establishments, and health clubs are beginning to install them.

Massage

When you're under stress, fight or flight hormones and waste substances can make your muscles tight to the point of pain. Without proper relaxation, these muscles can become chronically tight—particularly a problem in the neck, shoulders, and upper back. One of the most pleasant and effective ways of relieving muscular tension and lifting your spirits is having a massage.

• Shiatsu, from Japan and China, is a technique of deep massage of specific pressure points. In some cases, the Shiatsu masseuse may walk lightly on your back to work out hard knots.

• Swedish massage involves kneading and stroking the muscles to relax knots and improve blood circulation.

You don't have to go to a pro for a satisfying, beneficial massage. A willing spouse or friend can massage away some of your tension. (Lucky are those of us who have a friend at work who knows how to massage away a headache or a sore neck.) In a pinch, you can even massage yourself. Most people don't have much trouble reaching their neck and shoulders or legs and thighs.

Massage hints

1. A massage feels best when done with oil. Many stores sell special light massage oils. Baby oil or even something from the kitchen like peanut oil also works. The oil helps the massager's hands move easily over your skin without pulling it.

2. A heat lamp or hot towels can help loosen your muscles before a massage. This treatment also helps any trouble spots that you might have. If you have a sore lower back, for instance, you might want to apply these warm compresses or sit under a heat lamp several times a day. A heating pad that puts out moist heat may work better for you than dry heat for treating muscle spasms and tightness.

3. Many people like to listen to soothing music while they're being massaged.

4. You can work on knots of tension yourself by feeling along sore muscles until you get to a knot. The knot will hurt as you press it. Rub and knead the knot with a firm pressure, and rub the muscle as far as you can trace it in both directions. Repeat several times a day. This will help you release these painful spots.

How to give a relaxing back rub

Before starting, make sure your hands are warm and relaxed. Hold them under warm water or rub them together briskly. Since friction between your hands and the person's back may cause irritation, use lotion or oil to lubricate the person's skin (use a massage oil, baby oil, or olive, safflower, or peanut oil). Warm the lotion or oil first, either in your hands or by placing the bottle in warm water. Note: Use alcohol followed by powder if the person's skin is oily.

Starting at the base of the spine and using firm strokes, proceed upward to the person's shoulders. Rotate outward from the spine to include the entire back. Meanwhile, you may use the thumb and first three fingers of one hand to rub the person's shoulder or the nape of the neck.

Keeping both hands on the person's back at all times, make smooth transitions as you move from one stroke to another. This is more comfortable and relaxing than if you were to remove your hands and reapply them during the back rub.

To end the back rub, use long strokes up the length of the person's back, gradually reducing the pressure as you move your hands. These long, soothing strokes will bring further relaxation and comfort.

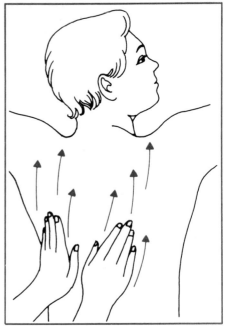

To begin a back rub, start at the base of the spine and work toward the shoulders.

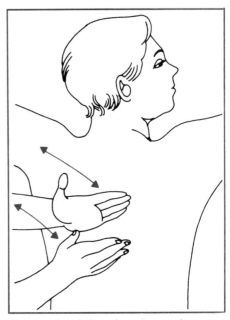

Use your hands in a chopping motion.

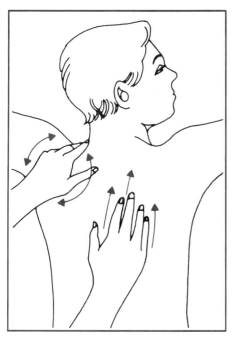

Use one hand to massage the person's shoulder or neck while you continue the back rub with your other hand.

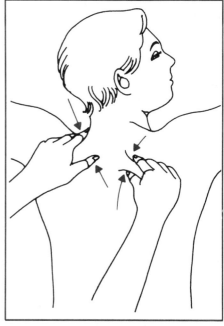

Grasp a portion of a muscle group in each hand and glide one hand toward the other as you squeeze.

As you rub and knead, feel for knots. Then concentrate on rubbing and kneading the knot and the muscles that lead to it and from it.

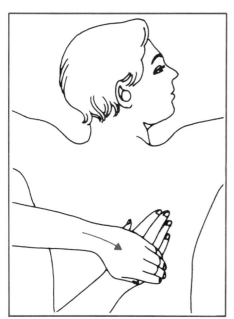

Place one hand on the other to reinforce pressure and make circles or transverse strokes.

Choosing the right activity

Aerobic exercise is the right choice for most people with hypertension. With aerobic effort, such as swimming, the muscles move naturally and rhythmically. To supply more oxygenated blood to the muscles as they work, the heart contracts more forcefully and the lungs expand more fully. As a result, the heart muscle becomes stronger.

Systolic blood pressure, which rises only slightly during the workout, may drop 25 percent or more after aerobic exercise. In time, a regular program of aerobic exercise can permanently lower at-rest blood pressure.

On the other hand, isometric exercise, such as weight lifting, is the wrong choice. Any exercise that involves sustained muscle contraction against resistance—pressing, squeezing, pushing, pulling, lifting—dramatically raises blood pressure. A professional weight lifter may experience blood pressure elevations as high as 450/300 during workouts. And the strain of even an everyday isometric effort like shoveling snow can quickly overwhelm a weakened cardiovascular system. Isometric exercises build bulk and strength, but they do little to strengthen the cardiovascular system—and that's what someone with hypertension needs to do.

Exercise

When you're in a fight or flight state, mobilized for action, you slowly exhaust all the systems of your body. If this sort of stress is kept up day after day without release, you're likely to set yourself up for a disease. The right kind of exercise done regularly can help you release your tensions and prevent disease. Exercise gives you an outlet for muscular tension caused by psychological stress. It also increases your body's efficiency in using oxygen, thus allowing your heart to work less hard to nourish your cells. And it can lower triglyceride and cholesterol levels and blood pressure. Exercise can also increase the activity of various anti-clotting agents in your blood. Since heart attacks and strokes may be caused by such clots being deposited on the walls of your arteries, this anti-clotting effect of exercise is also a boon to your good health. If done faithfully, exercise will also help keep your weight under control, which may help lower your risk of heart disease, hypertension, and diabetes. Incidentally, you may find that you also cut out some bad habits. After you've been smoking cigarettes all day, you'll find running more effortful. Give up the smoking! And you'll probably want to eat a better diet to give yourself more energy to exercise.

Exercise, like any sort of good or bad stress, causes the release of endorphins, our bodies' natural painkilling substances. The pituitary secretes endorphins along with ACTH, a hormone that triggers the release of the adrenal stress hormones. This ACTH released during the beneficial stress of hard exercise causes the release of epinephrine, which can make us feel tense and anxious or energetic and happy. Released during times of stress, it has a negative effect. It makes our blood pressure rise and our hearts pound. But when it's released during exercise, we work off the negative physical effects of epinephrine but still feel the euphoric psychological effects of both epinephrine and the endorphins. Incidentally, this may be one of the reasons that people often give up cigarettes when they begin a serious exercise program. Both smoking and exercise cause endorphin release. Some people may be able to switch over and get their endorphin "fix" from exercise rather than from cigarettes.

Aerobic exercise

In order to be effective, and especially to cause endorphin release, exercise should be aerobic and should be done often. (Naturally, you should check with your doctor before beginning any sort of exercise program.) Aerobic exercise is the kind that increases your breathing rate and makes your heart and lungs work. When doing an aerobic exercise, your goal is to get your heart to work at 70 percent of its maximum capacity and keep it there for 20 minutes. (Aerobic exercise shouldn't get you out of breath. A good rule of thumb for determining how hard you should do an aerobic exercise is that you should be able to hold a conversation at the same time. If you're too out of breath to do this, you're working too hard.) You should repeat your aerobics at least three times a week. Good aerobic exercises are fast walking, running, cycling, rowing, swimming, and cross-country skiing.

Types of exercises

Aerobic exercises	Isometric exercises	Combination aerobic and isometric exercises
Walking briskly	Weight lifting	Pulling a heavy cart
Jogging	Waterskiing	Carrying bundles
Running	Opening stuck	Wrestling
Push-ups	windows or jar lids	
Swimming	Pushing any immov-	
Bicycling	able object	
Shoveling		
Cross-country skiing		
Dancing		
Moving furniture		
Climbing stairs		
Handball		
Racquetball		
Soccer		
Sawing hardwood		

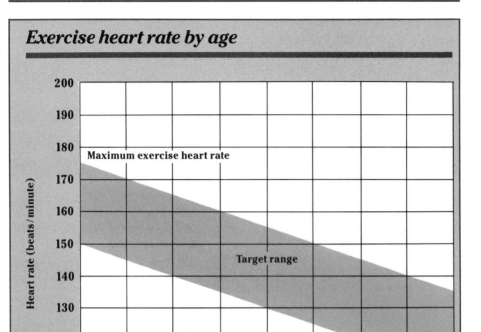

Exercise heart rate by age

To monitor your exercise program, determine your target heart rate and heart rate range. To calculate your target heart rate and target heart rate range, follow these steps:

• Subtract your age from 220. This is your maximum attainable heart rate —the highest rate at which your heart can work. If your age is 40, for example, your maximum heart rate is 180. (This calculation is based on the assumption that a person's heart rate declines by 1 beat/minute for each year he or she lives.)

• Calculate 75 percent of your maximum rate to determine your target heart rate. For example, if your maximum rate is 180, your target rate is 135 beats/minute. By maintaining this heart rate during exercise, you'll work your heart at 75 percent of its capacity—the ideal amount for cardiovascular fitness.

• To determine target heart rate range, calculate the range between 70 percent and 85 percent of your maximum heart rate. This calculation provides for the fact that people of the same age may have different resting heart rates. Don't exceed your target range. Refer to the chart for examples of target heart ranges according to age.

Monitor your heart rate

How can you check your heart rate? First, get a watch with a second hand. Then, as soon as you stop exercising, take your pulse in one of these two ways:

• Place your index and middle fingers on your wrist just below the thumb, as shown. (Don't use your thumb—it has a strong pulse of its own, which may confuse you.)

• If you have trouble feeling your wrist pulse, try this: place your thumb on your collarbone and lay your fingers along the side of your throat, as shown. You'll feel a strong pulse in your neck.

No matter which method you use, count the pulse beats for 6 seconds; then, add a zero to that figure. This gives you a reliable estimate of your working heart rate for 1 minute. (Don't count your pulse for a whole minute. Because your heart rate slows quickly when you rest, that figure won't be reliable.)

If your working heart rate is 10 beats or more above your target heart rate, don't work so hard the next time. But if your working heart rate is lower than your target rate, work a little harder next time. For instance, if you walk, walk faster—or even jog, if your doctor approves.

Why exercise?

Here's a checklist of common exercise benefits:
• *release tension*
• *improve sleep*
• *increase heart efficiency*
• *lower triglyceride and cholesterol levels*
• *lower blood pressure*
• *control weight*
• *decrease overall risk of heart attack*

Using exercise

If you aren't able to exert yourself in one of these very active sports for medical reasons such as rheumatoid arthritis, extreme obesity, or severe emphysema, a pleasant walk out of doors, a regular swim, or a ride on a stationary bicycle might be a more appropriate type of exercise, and any such exercise will bring you many benefits. Try to give yourself this break every day or every other day, weather permitting. Walking with a friend helps you make a habit of it, although you might want to walk alone with your thoughts some of the time, too.

For some people, exercise may be all you need to get yourself out of a mild to moderate depression caused by psychological stress. This is probably because exercise helps you to work off stress hormones that can make you feel tense and anxious or depressed. Exercise also helps you to stay more relaxed. A University of Wisconsin psychiatrist and runner, Dr. John Griest, put depressed patients on a 10-week walking and jogging program. Six out of the eight patients felt much better and stayed that way.

Use exercise as a way to break up your day. When you're frustrated with or tired of a particular task, take a break, get some exercise, and come back with a refreshed mind. Dr. Selye, who introduced the concept of stress to medicine, wrote: "Often a voluntary change of activity is as good as or even better than rest. When fatigue or enforced interruption prevents us from finishing a mathematical problem, it is better to go for a swim than simply sit around. Substituting demands made on our musculature for those previously made on the intellect not only gives our brain a rest, but helps us avoid worrying about the frustrating interruption. Stress on one system helps us to relax another."

Diet

Eating to counteract stress means avoiding those foods that are stressful for your body to process in excess. Such foods include those with many artificial additives, those that are salty, and those to which you're allergic. Eat instead those that are especially nourishing, and replace some of the vitamins and minerals that your body loses under stress. Include vegetables and a salad when you can.

Our American diet has gotten more and more estranged from what people ate just a generation or two ago. The American Heart Association and other organizations have urged us to revise some of our eating habits by limiting our intake of animal fats and salt. Excessive dietary fat plays an important role in atherosclerosis and heart disease and possibly also in breast and stomach and intestinal cancers. Too much sugar can push diabetes-prone individuals into full-blown diabetes, and too much salt can cause hypertension in salt-sensitive individuals.

(Text continued on page 88.)

Food additives

Much of the food we eat is processed, packed, and shipped far from where we live. The large companies that manufacture these mass-produced foods add numerous chemicals in order to color, preserve, stabilize, or flavor the food. Many of these chemicals are unnecessary, and many, although recognized as safe by the Food and Drug Administration, may not actually be so safe for everyone.

Coloring agents are the most widely used food additives. Although some foods are colored with harmless vegetable dyes, many more are colored with chemicals. As more is learned about what these chemicals do to the body, more are banned. For instance, the violet dye, Violet No. 1, that used to be used to stamp inspection seals on meats was banned in 1973 because it causes cancer. Red dye No. 4 is banned in everything except maraschino cherries because it harms the bladders and adrenal glands of dogs.

Sodium nitrite is a much-talked-about chemical used to flavor and color cured meats (and, until the late 1970s, even baby foods). Although sodium nitrite itself isn't thought to cause cancer, it combines with stomach chemicals to produce compounds known as nitrosamines, and these have caused cancer in laboratory animals. Manufacturers add sodium nitrite to such foods as cold cuts and bacon because people are accustomed to the artificial colors and cured tastes of these foods. (Many types of so-called hickory-smoked bacon have never been exposed to hickory smoke. The taste is artificial.)

Tips for successful low-fat dieting

- *When shopping, read product labels for fat content (or cholesterol content, if given). Buy only foods made with polyunsaturated or vegetable fats.*
- *Drink skim milk and use skim milk products.*
- *Follow your doctor's recommendation for the number of egg yolks you can safely eat each week.*

- *Limit your intake of beef, ham, and pork. Replace them with poultry, fish, or veal.*
- *Trim off as much fat from meat as possible before cooking it. Remove all poultry skin.*
- *Don't fry foods. Sauté food without butter in a nonstick frying pan. Or, use margarine or a nonstick vegetable oil spray.*

- *If you boil or simmer meat, immediately remove it from the cooking liquid when it's done.*
- *After preparing soups or gravies, chill them to allow the fat content to congeal; then skim off the fat before reheating and serving.*
- *Avoid creamy or cheesy sauces.*

Special note:
Read food labels when grocery shopping to determine an item's sodium content.

General eating guidelines

You probably feel that you don't have a lot of time to spend analyzing everything that you eat. Here are some general guidelines for healthful eating.

• Cut back on meats and other sources of fat. Meat is an excellent source of protein, but many of us eat too much to the point where fats begin to build up in our bloodstream. In many people, raised blood fats eventually lead to atherosclerosis, an important predisposing factor in heart disease, strokes, and some cases of hypertension. Cured meat is also high in salt.

Whole milk dairy products and many cheeses are high in fat. Choose skim milk over whole milk, and restrict your intake of cheese. Instead of using butter, you can use margarine or a vegetable oil. Most vegetable oils don't increase blood fats; some, such as safflower and sunflower oil, even help lower blood fats.

When you do eat meat, consider veal, which is lower in fat than beef, lamb, or pork. Trim away as much fat as you can, and broil the meat or cook it in a nonstick pan. Or eat fowl—chicken, duck, or turkey. (Incidentally, rabbit and venison are much lower in fat than any of the other meats listed here.)

• Cut back on refined sugars. Your body's cells burn sugars for fuel, but this doesn't mean you ever have to eat candy, cake, or ice cream. When you eat a candy bar, you may feel a temporary energy boost as your blood sugar level rises rapidly. Then your pancreas steps in and releases the hormone insulin, which removes the sugar from your blood and helps get it to the liver, where it's stored in a form usable by the body. Insulin's job is to make sure that you have the right amount of sugar in your blood for use by your cells.

The more refined the sugar, the more insulin release it provokes, because the refined sugars such as those found in candy are more easily broken down by your body and enter the bloodstream rapidly and all together. This rapid increase in blood sugar stimulates a stepped up insulin release to lower your blood sugar again. Sometimes excess insulin is released. When this happens, you feel fatigued, dizzy, cranky, and hungry for more sugar —signs that your blood sugar is low.

Your body has a better source of usable sugars in fruits, grains, nuts, pasta, and potatoes—so-called complex carbohydrates. The sugars in these foods are broken down more slowly during digestion, reach your bloodstream more gradually, and stimulate a steadier insulin release. Not only does this help keep you on a more even keel, but it also avoids stressing the pancreas with demands for bursts of insulin release, a process that some doctors believe may sometimes cause adult diabetes.

• Eat more fish. Not only is it lower in fat and calories, it contains eichosapentaenoic acid—better known as EPA—a type of fat that seems to lower blood fats and thus the risk of heart attacks. Such fish as salmon, mackerel, and tuna are particularly high in EPA.

• Cut back on salt. Americans consume many times the amount of salt that their bodies need to function healthily. As we've seen, excess salt may be a major culprit in many cases of hypertension, as well as premenstrual syndrome and migraine headaches.

You can reduce the salt in your diet by eating fewer processed foods. Fresh fruits and vegetables that are frozen without special sauces are low in salt. By comparison, one serving of canned peas or asparagus from a glass jar contains 255 times the salt found in fresh or frozen peas. Don't put the salt shaker on the table, and don't add salt during cooking; rely instead on seasonings such as garlic, lemon juice, and herbs and spices. Although you may crave salt at first, if you slowly cut down, you'll find that your desire for salt will disappear within a couple of months. You'll find that you'll be able to taste the salt that naturally occurs in meats,

vegetables, grains, and dairy products. Processed foods will begin to taste over-salted to you, and you'll have no trouble staying away from them.

• Eat more fresh fruits and vegetables. Not only do they provide you with many vitamins and minerals, but they also provide fiber to help keep your intestines functioning well. Beta carotene, the form of Vitamin A found in many vegetables and fruits, may help protect us against certain types of cancer. While this protection hasn't been proven, many doctors are now urging their patients to step up their ingestion of these foods. Vitamin C and bioflavonoids help keep your blood vessels strong, too.

• Eat more whole grains. Taking the hull off grains such as rice to make them white and quicker to cook is a nutritional mistake. The hulls contain the highest concentration of nutrients. They also provide fiber, which helps keep your intestines healthy and may play a role in clearing excess fats from your blood.

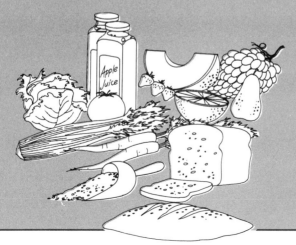

Time management

No matter who you are or what your occupation, you're probably busy. Insufficient time seems to be a fact of late 20th century life. How well you manage your time may play a large role in deciding how much pressure you feel.

- Are you always running late?

- Do you feel that you always have too much to do?

- Do you feel guilty about time taken off from work?

- Do you feel guilty at the time work takes from your home life?

- Do you put things off?

- Do you routinely work weekends?

- Do you have trouble saying no?

"Yes" answers to these questions indicate that you may need some help managing your time to minimize stress. Although the question of time management is big enough for a large book of its own, here are some tips:

- Many people who can never seem to find time need to set goals for themselves. If you don't know what you really want, you won't know what to do first. Make a list of your goals. Where do you want to be next year? In five, ten years? This doesn't mean that you have to set yourself on some irrevocable course, but having definite long-term goals will help you make choices about how to spend your time now.

- Learn how to set priorities. Not everything that you have to do is equally important. When you have thought out your goals, you'll be halfway toward knowing what your priorities should be.

- You may not always have a great deal of choice whether you work overtime. But some people must work overtime because they aren't disciplined enough to get their work done on time. Learn how to stop being inefficient. Self-hypnosis can be a valuable tool to help you discipline your work habits. Tell yourself that you will work hard during work hours and that you will not work or think about work in the evenings or on the weekends. Keep this separation in your life.

Aromatherapy

Things that smell good may help relieve anxiety, headaches, hypertension, and other stress-related disorders. Natural healers and so-called aromatherapists have existed for years. Now aromas are of interest in more accredited medical circles. Gary Schwartz, MD, professor of psychiatry and psychology at Yale University, uses the healing power of scent in the treatment of many diseases and disorders.

Of all the scents he has tested to reduce stress, a spicy apple scent reminiscent of cider or apple pie seems to work best. In one study, the spicy apple fragrance caused subjects' systolic blood pressure (the upper reading) to fall by three to four points.

You might experiment to see which scents work for you. Some people find that rose oil is very calming and that peppermint or lavender oil is stimulating. If you do respond to a particular scent, why not keep a small vial with you to bring out whenever you need a pick-me-up?

• Learn to say no. Too often we get suckered into saying we'll take on more work than we know we can handle just because we want to please the other person. Remember that your first need is to do the job at hand well, not to take on too much work and do a rushed, under-par job. Be polite but firm about your other time commitments.

• Take off brief quiet times during the day when you let the cares of work slide from your shoulders for five minutes. You might want to get up and move around, even go outside if you can. These five-minute breaks are also excellent times to practice some of the techniques discussed earlier in this chapter.

Time-out

As much as you need routine to keep your life running smoothly, you also need time away from the routine to rest, regenerate, and even expand your horizons. Well-timed, planned vacations can be the very quickest stress reducers, because they can remove us immediately from the cares and hassles of our day-to-day lives. Although you might need a day or two of adjustment, you'll find that a change of scene or at least of routine can put your cares far behind you.

Whether you decide to stay around home or take a trip, remember that the point of a vacation is to let go and relax. Many people feel that they have to accomplish something while on vacation. Some run themselves off their feet sight-seeing, while others use that time to do all the yard and house work that they have been putting off all year. Either way, they're likely to return to work not refreshed but rather browned out. If you like to sight-see or want to put a few spare hours into cleaning up your garage for the lift it will give you when you're finished, then go ahead. But don't feel that you have to put your vacation time to definite use. Instead, try thinking of your vacation as a time to compensate for the rest of the year. If you've lived through a stressful year, you need time to rest and regenerate. Perhaps a week on a beach or a camping trip would help. If instead you've had an uneventful, routine sort of year, you might want to break radically with your routine for a couple of weeks. A trip to another country or state, or lessons in a new sport, might be just the ticket.

Too many things to do
What time is it? Where are you supposed to be? The day-to-day pressure of appointments, meetings, errands, chores, and bits of information to remember can lead to stress. If you can't change your hectic schedule, try to change the way you approach your responsibilities and make use of the de-stressors described farther on.

The value of friendship

Friends may be the best medicine. Think how good you feel when you discuss problems with a friend or share an afternoon doing a sport that you both enjoy. If you don't have some close friends with whom you can share the joys and sorrows of life, you may be missing out on one of the most important (and healthy) experiences. Yet many of us feel that we don't have any close friends to turn to in time of need.

"I used to have a lot of friends in the town where I grew up, but I moved away from there eight years ago when I got married, and I never seem to have a chance to go back and visit them or even to call them up. Sometimes I'm very lonely here. Of course, I have my husband and the children, but sometimes I wish I had more time to hang out with friends the way I used to. I guess that's just the way life goes. Each year seems to

Recipe for a great vacation

1. Plan well ahead. Not only can you get better travel deals, but you'll also avoid wasting any of your precious vacation time wondering what to do.

2. Give yourself a day to disengage from the concerns of your work life and get oriented to vacation time. This is also the day to pack and close up your house if you're going away.

3. Neaten your work area and leave yourself a memo describing where your projects stand and reminding you where to pick up again after your vacation. Then forget your work. Don't take any work with you on vacation—even though this may be hard for you.

4. Give up control. Although you have to be in control while you're at work and in your daily routine, you can't be completely in control on any vacation that takes you away from home. Small things seem to go wrong on any vacation, but don't let these upset you. No one expects you to be in control. Go with the flow and see whether you can't take petty problems like lost reservations and missed trains as the doorway to adventure, not as more hassles.

Relationships matter

Unhappy people often succumb to illness. How can you avoid unhappiness? One proven way is to work at friendships, emotional ties, and love. Those who outlive a spouse can still give and receive affection with friends, relatives, and even pets. Not surprisingly, unmarried people in loving relationships are healthier as a group than unhappily married ones. If you need affection, try new friends — or buy a pet.

get busier and busier." This woman's complaint is extremely common. In today's world so many of us feel too busy or even too tired for friendship—even though we may be longing for it. New research is showing that we may pay a price for ignoring this important part of our lives. Exercise, diet, and good medical care are of course very important to our health, but good health depends on more than these measures. Personal relationships are very important. Spouses, family members, friends, and even pets can contribute to our health and happiness.

Having someone on your side at home really helps. A study of 10,000 male Israeli civil servants found that men who described their wives as loving and supportive had a much lower incidence of angina than men who didn't have such a relationship. This was true even for men with physical and psychological factors that put them at a higher risk of developing heart disease.

Happy marriages are very important in maintaining psychological and bodily health, but the benefit may come from having a confidant, whether or not you're married to that person. One study found that married people generally reported greater satisfaction with life than did people whose spouses had died. This was to be expected, but the study also found that widowed people with a close confidant were happier than married people who felt that they didn't have anyone to confide in.

Bonds with other people play an important role in keeping us healthy. A twenty-year ongoing study of 7,000 residents of Alameda County, California, found that people who didn't have any close emotional bonds had a two to five times higher death rate than those who did have important, sustaining relationships. Amazingly, the study showed that ties to other people were more important in determining who would get sick or die than drinking, smoking, obesity, and exercise.

Depression and other emotional disorders can be caused by a lack of friends, but how do you explain the higher rates of heart disease and certain types of cancer among people who don't have significant relationships in their lives? Perhaps the immune system doesn't function up to par if you're lonely and have no one to turn to. Doctors have found that various immune system agents are suppressed when you're depressed, so that you have less ability to fight off harmful invaders.

You may have found that being a good friend or keeping good friends is difficult. Jobs and marriage often bring relocation, new responsibilities, and an end to the daily sessions with your friends. Even after assembling a compatible circle of friends, many couples find that child raising changes all that. Somehow between work and being with the family, you might have little time left for friends—unless you make time.

Sleep

Although some experiments indicate that we may get as much rest as we need from a half-hour float or meditation session, we still need to sleep and dream. How much sleep should you get? Most doctors agree that somewhere around eight hours is a good average. Some people need only six or seven hours while oth-

The magic of laughter

Laughter and positive emotions may play an important part in helping you get well and stay well. The famous story of Norman Cousins, a well-known writer and magazine editor, is a case in point. Cousins was diagnosed as having a disease of the connective tissues of his body. He was in so much pain all the time that, "To move your thumbs was like walking on your eyeballs." His doctors told him that he had a one in 500 chance of a full recovery and pumped him with 26 aspirin tablets each day plus other anti-inflammatory drugs and painkillers.

Cousins, who had some medical knowledge, felt that the drugs were making him worse. His doctor tested him and found that he was indeed extremely sensitive to all the drugs he was receiving. With his doctor's permission, Cousins totally changed his treatment. On the theory that his body was not getting the rest it needed in the hospital environment, he moved to a nearby hotel. He substituted large doses of Vitamin C for the drugs and ordered up a slew of movies—re-runs of "Candid Camera" and the Marx Brothers. Despite the intense pain, he began to laugh uproariously. Then something verging on the miraculous began to happen. The more he laughed, he realized, the less pain he noticed. "Ten minutes of belly laughter gave me an hour of pain-free sleep....The more I laughed, the better I got."

The point of this story is not to suggest that you should defy your doctor's orders and try to medicate yourself, but to indicate once again the power of positive emotions in influencing your health. Put simply: you have a choice of how to respond to illness and pain. Try to smile or laugh and you'll find that not only do you feel better on the spot but that your body will recover faster.

Here are some tips on making and maintaining friendships:

• *Think about what you want from your friends and then try to be that sort of person too.*

• *Go places and do things. Good places to meet friends: mixers, volunteer work, jobs, churches, sports, and lectures.*

• *If you meet someone you like, don't let the person escape. Make a date on the spot to have lunch or dinner.*

• *Have a party to meet your neighbors.*

• *Don't just say, "Let's have lunch sometime." Get out your date book and schedule your friends in.*

ers don't feel their best unless they have had nine. If you're routinely sleeping more than ten hours, you have a clue that you're under a lot of stress and that your body needs more sleep than usual. Oversleeping can also be a sign of depression. While you'll probably sleep less as you age, if you're sleeping only four or five hours and feel tired from lack of sleep, you may also be suffering from the effects of stress and its attendant anxiety. Here are some suggestions for helping you fall asleep and stay asleep.

• Don't go to bed with worries. You can always think about your problems tomorrow if a good night's sleep hasn't sorted them out for you. In the meantime, do yourself a favor and put them out of your mind. Meditation, biofeedback, or self-hypnosis can all help you do this if you routinely go to bed with your mind tumbling over and over like a washing machine.

• Don't get revved up by exercising near bedtime, but a quiet walk around the block with the dog or a few minutes of star gazing might be a restful way to put an end to the day.

• Exercise during the day can work out your muscles enough to make you sleep better at night.

• Some people find that reading helps them slide into a good sleep.

• Take a warm, but not hot, bath before you go to bed to relax your mind and muscles.

• A cup of warm milk before you go to bed may make you feel pleasantly drowsy.

• If you occasionally can't fall asleep or you wake up in the middle of the night, don't get upset and worried. Get up for a few minutes and read until you're drowsy again. If it's not too early, you might get up and go out for a morning adventure.

Index